This book is a synopsis

of the larger book,

"Understanding

Diabetes,"

11th edition.

It provides a quick summary

of each of the 28 chapters.

It may be easier to begin

learning from this book

until you are ready

to read the larger book.

# A FIRST BOOK FOR UNDERSTANDING DIABETES

COMPANION TO THE 11TH EDITION
OF "UNDERSTANDING DIABETES"

## H. Peter Chase, MD

BARBARA DAVIS CENTER FOR CHILDHOOD DIABETES
DEPARTMENT OF PEDIATRICS
UNIVERSITY OF COLORADO AT DENVER
AND HEALTH SCIENCES CENTER

PUBLISHED BY
CHILDREN'S DIABETES FOUNDATION
AT DENVER

For information, contact

Children's Diabetes Foundation at Denver
777 Grant Street, Suite 302
Denver, CO 80203

www.ChildrensDiabetesFoundation.org


Chase, H. Peter.
    A first book for understanding diabetes : companion
to the 11th edition / H. Peter Chase.
    p. cm.
    LCCN 2007920717
    ISBN-13: 978-0-9815381-5-0
    ISBN-10: 0-9815381-5-0

    1. Diabetes--Popular works.    I. Chase, H. Peter.
Understanding diabetes.  II. Title.

RC660.4.C43 2008                616.4'62
                                QBI07-600072


Please direct questions to:
Hilton Publishing Company
1630 45th Street, Suite 103    Munster, IN  46321
    219-922-4868    www.hiltonpub.com


Book Design by Scott Johnson


Printed in the United States of America

1  3  5  7  9  10  8  6  4  2

# FOREWORD

These ten fingers are all I have and I need them for my work so I'm very careful about treating my diabetes! If I can test my blood sugar without having to hurt myself, well then that's a good day, I think. At 83 years old, I have refused to let diabetes slow me down and I take my health very seriously, as you should for your whole life.

I've had type 2 diabetes for 25 years and I've put the same energy into staying healthy that I do with my music. I don't eat sweets much and avoid sugar. I'm a careful eater, love fish and a little meat, so I don't have any real bad problems. I guess I don't do EVERYTHING I should—it wouldn't be any fun if we didn't cautiously sneak a sweet once in a while!

Some days, I don't even feel like I have diabetes, now that's amazing! When I got a diagnosis it came as a surprise. I didn't know much about diabetes. After learning I can control diabetes in my life I began to radiate more confidence. It's fairly easy to have a balanced life with diabetes, but it wasn't always that way.

I hope my presence and what I say will encourage someone and help them learn the truth about diabetes and what to do about it. Some folks don't think that diabetes can be life-threatening. But that's incorrect. I lost close family members who had diabetes. Make sure you regularly check your blood sugar and see your doctor.

I've been able to stick to a daily routine by managing my diabetes. Blood glucose testing has become much easier over the years, and I test every day. I've also learned how to shop. I can go buy sugar-free candy and ice cream and cookies. I don't eat a lot of heavy foods and I try to eat vegetables quite often, and not too many fattening foods. Good luck and remember to learn as much as you can about diabetes and put it to good use in your life, it's all in this book.

By doing the right thing, you can have a long and fulfilling life!

B.B. KING

This book is dedicated to
Dr. George Eisenbarth
who has done such an excellent job
as the Center's third Executive Director.

# SPECIAL THANKS TO...

- The staff of the Children's Diabetes Foundation and The Guild of the Children's Diabetes Foundation at Denver.

- Proof-readers Kate Bostick, Lisa Fisher and Alice Hower.

- Regina Reece for manuscript preparation, editing and proofreading.

- Scott Johnson for book design, graphics, and illustrations.

- MGM Consumer Products for allowing the use of The Pink Panther™.
  www.pinkpanther.com

- Additional copies of this publication may be purchased from the Children's Diabetes Foundation at Denver. See available publications at the end of this book.

# Table of Contents

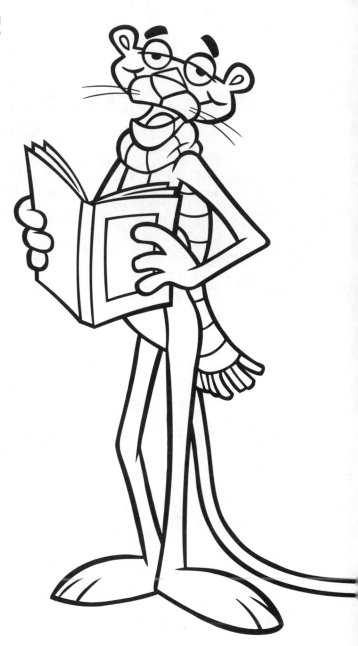

Chapter 1    The Importance of
             Education in Diabetes          1

Chapter 2    What is Diabetes?             5

Chapter 3    What Causes
             Type 1 Diabetes?              9

Chapter 4    Type 2 Diabetes
             (Non-Insulin Dependent
             Diabetes Mellitus [NIDDM])   11

Chapter 5    Ketone Testing               13

Chapter 6    Low Blood Sugar
             (Hypoglycemia or
             Insulin Reaction)            15

Chapter 7    Blood Sugar
             (Glucose) Testing            21

Chapter 8    Insulin:
             Types and Activity           25

Chapter 9    Drawing Up Insulin
             and Insulin Injections       31

Chapter 10   Feelings and Diabetes        37

Chapter 11   Normal Nutrition             39

Chapter 12   Food Management
             and Diabetes                 41

Chapter 13   Exercise and
             Diabetes                     45

Chapter 14   Diabetes and
             Blood Sugar Control          49

Chapter 15  Ketonuria and Acidosis
            (Diabetic Ketoacidosis
            or DKA)             53

Chapter 16  Sick-day and Surgery
            Management          59

Chapter 17  Family Concerns     67

Chapter 18  Responsibilities
            of Children at
            Different Ages      71

Chapter 19  Special Challenges
            of the Teen Years   75

Chapter 20  Outpatient
            Management, Education,
            Support Groups, and
            Standards of Care   79

Chapter 21  Adjusting the Insulin
            Dose, Correction Factors,
            and "Thinking" Scales  83

Chapter 22  Long-term Complications
            of Diabetes         87

Chapter 23  The School
            and Diabetes        91

Chapter 24  Baby-sitters,
            Grandparents, and
            Other Caregivers    97

Chapter 25  Vacations and
            Camp                101

Chapter 26  Use of Insulin Pumps
            in Diabetes
            Management          105

Chapter 27  Pregnancy and
            Diabetes            109

Chapter 28  Research and
            Diabetes            111

Author Bio/Disclosure           115

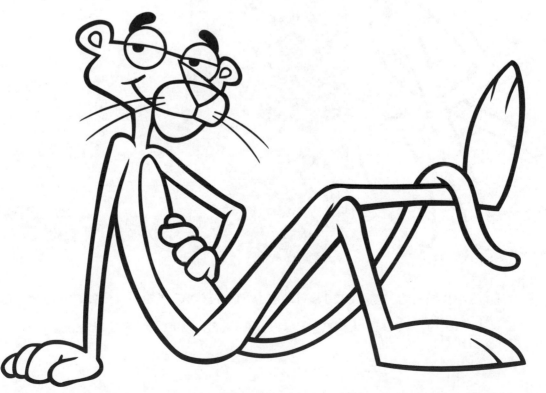

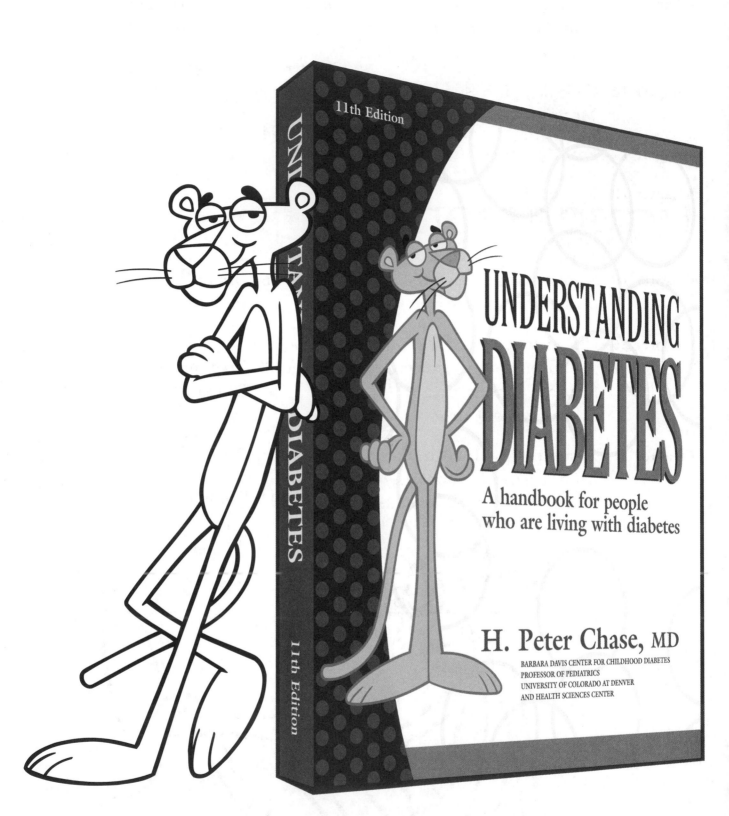

The Chapters in this book follow the chapters in
"Understanding Diabetes," 11th edition.

# Chapter 1
# The Importance of Education in Diabetes

H. Peter Chase, MD
DeAnn Johnson, RN, BSN, CDE

It is important to learn all about diabetes. At the time of diagnosis the family will spend two to three days learning about diabetes. A week later they will return for another day. This book will help in the beginning, until the family is ready to read "Understanding Diabetes." In both books, the chapters have the same numbers and topics. All family members, including both parents, should be present for initial education.

🐾 The **first** day of teaching often includes:

☐ What diabetes is and what causes it
☐ Urine and/or blood ketone testing
☐ Blood sugar testing
☐ Recognizing a low blood sugar and how to treat it
☐ Insulin types and actions
☐ Drawing up insulin
☐ Giving shots
☐ Food survival skills

🐾 On the **second** day, the topics from day one are reviewed and a family member gives the shot. Other areas often covered are:

☐ A school plan
☐ Directions for diabetes care using the telephone
☐ Details of treatment (including "thinking" scales)
☐ Education about food (dietitian)
☐ Feelings (psych-social team)
☐ Plans for the next few days

🐾 **One-Week** Follow Up

Usually at one-week the family and child return for more education with other families. The content includes: teaching done by the dietitian and nurse and a clinic visit with the physician. Areas covered include:

☐ Details of food management with diabetes
☐ Review of $HbA_{1c}$: what is it, why is it important

- ☐ Insulin actions and different insulin regimens
- ☐ Pattern management of blood sugars: how to identify trends and when to fax or e-mail numbers (all families are given fax sheets to send in weekly for at least four to six weeks)
- ☐ Low blood sugar care: causes, signs and treatment of mild to severe low blood sugars including a review of the use of glucose tablets and gel, honey, and administration of glucagon

- ☐ High blood sugar care: prevention of diabetic ketoacidosis; causes, signs and treatment
- ☐ Sick-day management: how often to check blood sugar and ketones, fluid replacement, what type and how much, when and how to urgently call for assistance

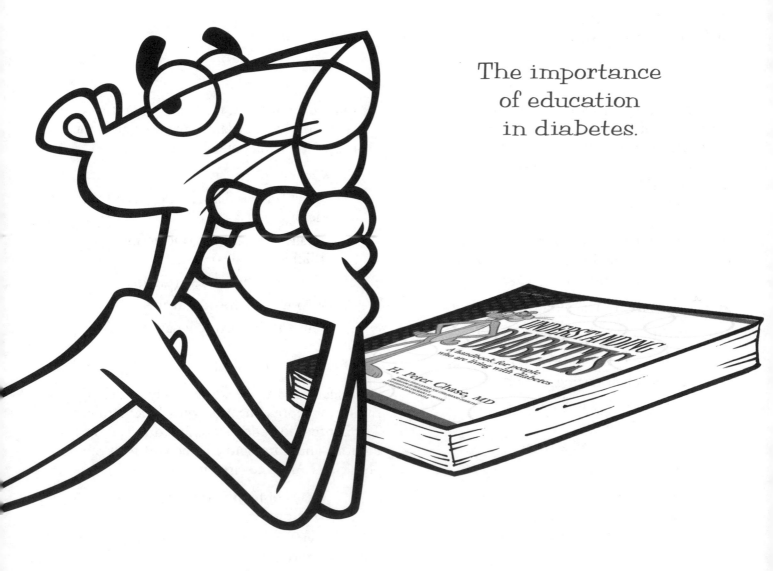

The importance of education in diabetes.

# Special Instructions for the first night are:

New Patient First-Night Instructions for _____

**A.** *The diabetes supplies you will need the first night include* (your nurse will mark which you need):

| | | |
|---|---|---|
| ____ Blood glucose meter | ____ Meter test strips | ____ Alcohol swabs |
| ____ Ketone check strips | ____ Glucose gel & tabs | ____ Log book |
| ____ Insulin | ____ Syringes | ____ Phone contact card |

The first night you will either get your insulin injection at our clinic, or you will give the shot at home or where you are staying.

**B.** *If the insulin is given while at the clinic:*

☐ 1. Humalog®/NovoLog®/Apidra® insulin has been given; eat within 10-15 minutes.

☐ 2. Regular insulin has been given, try to eat your meal within 30 minutes – or – have a snack containing carbohydrates on the way home if it will be more than 30 minutes.

☐ 3. Allow your child to eat until their appetite is satisfied, avoiding high sugar foods (especially regular sugar pop [soda] and sweet desserts).

**C.** *If the dinner insulin is to be given at home:*

1. Check your child's blood sugar right before your meal. Enter the result into the log book.

2. Check for urine ketones. Enter the result into the log book.

3. Call Dr. _____ at _____ or page at _____ for an insulin dose.

   *Give this dose:* _____.

4. Draw up and give the insulin injection right before your meal (see Chapter 8). If your child is not very hungry or is tired, you can give the shot after they eat and call the physician with any dose questions.

5. Eat your meal, allowing your child to eat until their appetite is satisfied. Avoid high sugar foods.

**D.** *Before Bed:*

1. Check your child's blood sugar. Enter the result into the log book.

2. Check for urine ketones. Enter the result into the log book.

3. Call your physician at the numbers listed above if your child's blood sugar is below ____ or above ____, or if urine ketones are "moderate" or "large." If urine ketones are "trace" or "small," have your child drink 8-12 oz of water before going to bed.

4. Give an insulin injection if your physician instructs you to do so. (Dose, if ordered = _____.)

5. Have your child eat a bedtime snack. Some ideas for this snack include: cereal and milk, toast and peanut butter, a slice of pizza, yogurt and graham crackers, or cheese and crackers. (See Chapter 11, Table 2 in the *Understanding Diabetes* book for other ideas.)

**E.** *The second morning before coming to the clinic:*

1. If your physician has instructed you to give the morning insulin at home before coming in, follow the steps listed above (see letter **"C"**) for last night's meal dose **before** eating breakfast.

2. If you have been instructed to wait to give the morning dose until after coming to the clinic, do a blood sugar test and a urine ketone test upon awakening (if blood sugar is less than 70 mg/dl [3.9 mmol/L], give 4–6 oz of juice promptly).

   Write the blood sugar and urine ketone results in your log book.
   ☐ Eat breakfast at home, and then come to the clinic for your insulin injection.
   ☐ Bring your breakfast to the clinic, and you will eat it after the insulin has been given.

3. Please bring all blood testing supplies and materials you received the first day back to the clinic (including your log book, Pink Panther book, insulin and supplies).

Insulin is made in the body by
an organ called the pancreas.
The difference between people
with type 1 diabetes and
people with type 2 diabetes
is the pancreas of a person
with type 1 diabetes stops
making enough insulin.

In type 2 diabetes,
the pancreas can still make
insulin, but the insulin does
not work like it should.

Esophagus

Heart

Stomach

Intestine

Pancreas

Kidneys

Bladder

# Chapter 2
# What Is Diabetes?

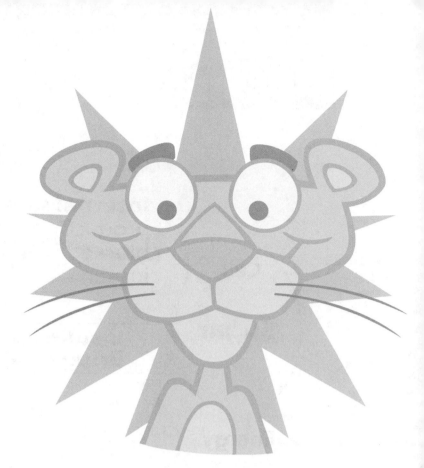

**Type 1** (Childhood, Juvenile, Insulin-dependent) **diabetes** is due to not enough insulin being made in the pancreas (see picture). The most common signs arc:

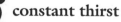 **1** **frequent passing of urine**

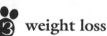 **2** **constant thirst**

**3** **weight loss**

For people with **type 1 diabetes**, insulin must be taken through a needle. Insulin cannot be taken as a pill because the stomach acid would destroy it.

Type 1 diabetes is different from **type 2 diabetes** (adult-onset, or non-insulin dependent diabetes) where insulin is still made but doesn't work very well. People with type 2 diabctcs can somctimcs use pills (which are not insulin) and diet and exercise to control their diabetes (see Chapter 4). Eating healthy food and exercising are also important for people with type 1 diabetes, but they will always need to take insulin shots.

Insulin allows sugar to pass into our cells to be used for energy. It also turns off the body's making of sugar. When not enough insulin is present, the sugar cannot pass into the body's cells. The sugar is high in the blood and it passes out in the urine. Frequent passing of urine is the result. (See Figures on the next 2 pages.)

Because sugar cannot be used for energy, the body breaks down fat for energy. Ketones are the result of using fat for energy.

When insulin treatment begins, the urine ketones (see Chapter 5) gradually disappear. After a few days, the blood sugars become lower and the passing of urine and drinking of water will be less often. Weight is gained back and the person starts to feel much better.

Often a **"honeymoon"** time begins a few weeks or months after a person with type 1 diabetes starts insulin shots. The insulin dose (amount of insulin given) may go down and it may seem like the person does not have diabetes, but **THEY DO!** This period may last from two weeks to two years.

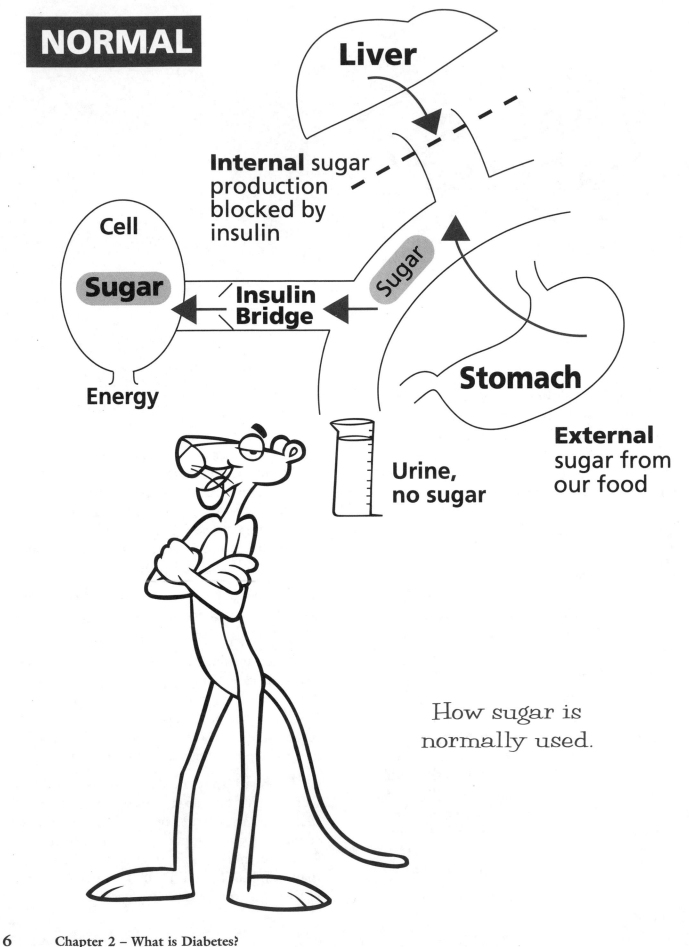

# NORMAL

**Liver**

**Internal** sugar production blocked by insulin

**Cell**

**Sugar**

**Energy**

**Insulin Bridge**

Sugar

**Stomach**

Urine, no sugar

**External** sugar from our food

How sugar is normally used.

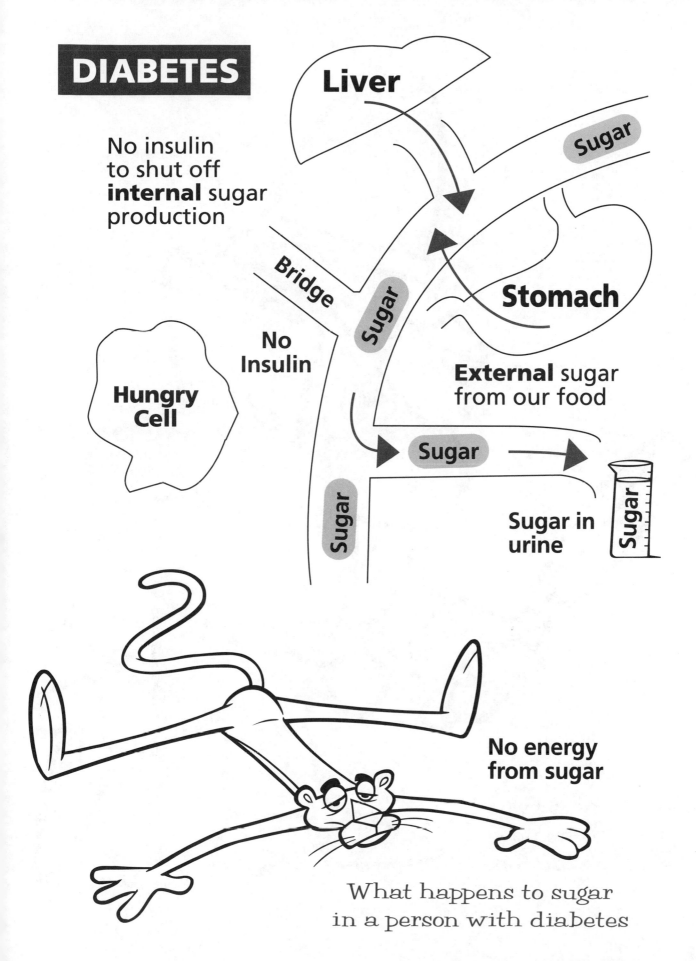

# DIABETES

**Liver**

No insulin to shut off **internal** sugar production

Sugar

Bridge

Sugar

No Insulin

**Stomach**

**Hungry Cell**

**External** sugar from our food

Sugar

Sugar

Sugar

Sugar in urine

No energy from sugar

What happens to sugar in a person with diabetes

The mystery of
what causes type 1
diabetes is now
better understood.

# Chapter 3
# What Causes Type 1 Diabetes?

The cause of type 1 diabetes is believed to be due to three things:

**①** **Genetics:** Genes come from both mom and dad and can make someone more likely to get diabetes. Over half of the people that get type 1 diabetes have inherited the gene cell types DR3/DR4. (One is from mom and one is from dad.)

**②** **Self-Allergy (autoimmunity):**

- The immune system in the body normally protects it from possible harm.

- An allergy is a reaction by the body's immune system to something it thinks doesn't belong inside the body.

- Self-allergy is when a person's body develops an allergy against one of its own parts. In this case, the allergy is against the islet (eye-let) cells in the pancreas where insulin is made. When the islet cells have been damaged, the immune system makes something called antibodies. These antibodies are present in the blood (**I**slet **C**ell **A**ntibodies or **ICA**).

Other antibodies that may be found in the blood of people with type 1 diabetes are:

- IAA (insulin autoantibody)
- GAD antibody
- ICA512 antibody

Sometimes these antibodies are present for many years before the signs of diabetes appear. Half of the people who will someday develop type 1 diabetes already have the antibodies by age five years. Being able to identify antibodies has allowed studies (which have begun in the U.S. and elsewhere) to try to prevent type 1 diabetes (see Chapter 28 on Research).

**③** **Virus or Chemical:** Having a certain gene makeup may allow a virus or chemical to get to the islet cells (where insulin is made) and cause damage. Once the damage has occurred, the self-allergy likely begins.

# TYPE 2 DIABETES

Type 2 (adult-onset) diabetes does not occur as a result of the self-allergy like type 1 diabetes.  Therefore, antibodies (found in type 1 diabetes) are not present in the blood.

Type 2 has an inherited part (Chapter 4), but the genetics are different from type 1 diabetes.  As noted in Chapter 2, people with type 2 diabetes may have normal or high insulin levels.  The insulin just does not work well.  In contrast, people with type 1 diabetes have low or no insulin.  The two conditions are both called diabetes.  Both result in high sugars, but they are VERY different from each other.

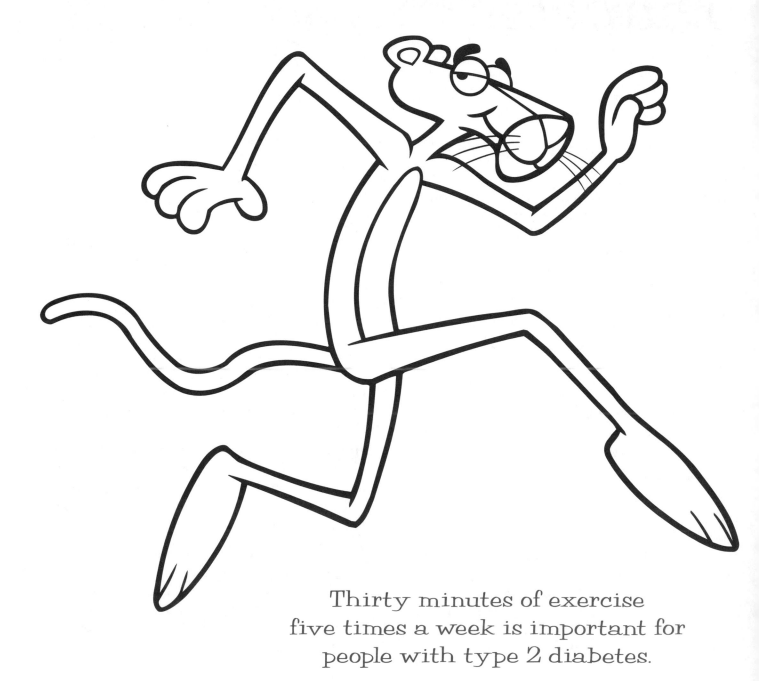

Thirty minutes of exercise
five times a week is important for
people with type 2 diabetes.

# Chapter 4
# Type 2 Diabetes

## (NON-INSULIN DEPENDENT DIABETES MELLITUS [NIDDM])

Type 2 diabetes is the most common type to occur in adults over age 40 years. It is also becoming more common in youth (particularly in overweight teenagers). It is quite common in Native-Americans. At least half of African-American and Hispanic youth with diabetes have type 2 diabetes.

## CAUSE

Type 2 diabetes is partly **inherited (genetic)**. It is also linked with being overweight and not getting enough exercise. It is often called a **"disease of life-styles."** Our ancestors were very active and ate less. We now live in a world of automobile travel, television, computers, video games, and high calorie fast foods.

## SYMPTOMS

The symptoms can be the same as with type 1 diabetes (Chapter 2). They may be:

 frequent drinking of liquids

 frequent urination (going to the bathroom)

 infections

 sores that heal slowly

 no energy

 Many people don't have any symptoms. These people are sometimes diagnosed by a high blood sugar that is measured on a routine physical exam. Others are diagnosed when they have a high blood sugar level on a test called an Oral Glucose Tolerance Test.

## TREATMENT: CHANGES IN LIFESTYLE ARE <u>VERY IMPORTANT</u>.

- Eating foods with fewer calories and carbohydrates as well as less fat is needed.

- Getting at least 30 minutes of exercise five to seven days a week is very important.

- Checking blood sugars (like people with type 1 diabetes) is helpful (Chapter 7). The blood sugar values can tell you how you are doing each day.

- If at diagnosis a person has ketones, insulin shots are usually needed. The shots are needed during times of illness.

- Medications by mouth can be tried if the blood sugars and HbA$_{1c}$ (Chapter 14) return to near normal. Often by losing weight and exercising, blood sugars will return to near normal.

- These medicines taken by mouth ARE NOT insulin. When taken, these medicines cause the pancreas to make more insulin. They can also make the body more sensitive to its own insulin.

  One of these medicines is called metformin (Glucophage®).

- This medicine is usually tried first.

- Sometimes it can cause an upset stomach.

- If a person becomes sick, this medicine must be stopped until they are well. It can cause a condition called lactic acidosis. Insulin shots may be needed during the illness. Call your doctor or nurse if you are not sure what to do.

- There are other medicines taken by mouth that can be tried if metformin causes too much stomach upset or isn't working well.

Testing
for
ketones.

# Chapter 5
# Ketone Testing

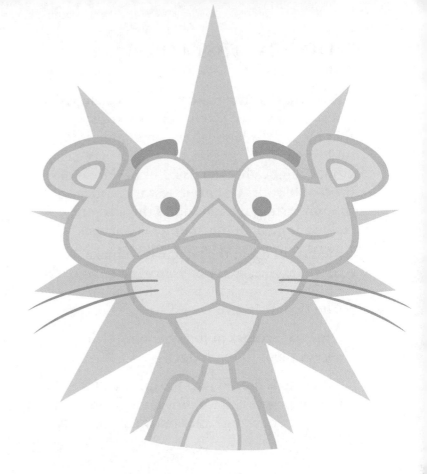

Ketone testing is very easy and very important.

## A. NEWLY DIAGNOSED PERSON:

**① The first goal for new patients is to clear their ketones.**

Ketones come from fat breakdown. Insulin stops fat breakdown and prevents ketones from being made.

**② The second goal is to lower their blood sugar levels.**

Insulin also turns off sugar production from the liver.

## B. A PERSON WITH KNOWN DIABETES:

**When to check for ketones (either in urine or blood):**

• during any illness

• with a very high blood sugar (e.g., above 300 mg/dl [16.7 mmol/L])

• if an insulin shot is missed

• after vomiting even once

• with a blockage of an insulin pump catheter or pump failure

If ketones are present, extra insulin can be given to stop the ketones from being made. (Ketones need to be found early and extra insulin given or the person may get very sick; see Chapter 15.)

## C. HOW TO TEST FOR KETONES

A method to test for ketones must always be in the home and taken along on trips. Failure to do the ketone test when indicated could result in the person becoming very sick. Ketones can be checked using either urine or a drop of blood. The urine test is cheaper, although testing the blood has the advantage of telling how high the ketones are at that moment (as well as other advantages).

### URINE TESTING

The two main strips used are:

1. Ketostix®: comes in foil wrapping that allows them to last longer.

   This strip is dipped into the urine and is read as negative, trace, small, moderate, large, or large-large after *exactly* 15 seconds.

2. Chemstrip K®: comes in bottles and are not foil wrapped. All non-foil wrapped strips (including non-foil wrapped Ketostix in a bottle) must be thrown out six months after the bottle is opened.

   This strip is dipped into the urine and is read as negative, trace, small, moderate, large or large-large after *exactly* 60 seconds.

### BLOOD TESTING

Some people prefer to use the Precision Xtra® meter to test blood ketones.

- The red calibration strip must be placed in the meter first.

- Next, the blood ketone strip is inserted with the three black bars facing up.

- Then a drop of blood is placed in the purple hole of the strip.

- The result is given in about 10 seconds.

Table
## Comparison of Blood and Urine Ketone Readings

| Blood Ketone (mmol/L) | Urine Ketone | | Action to take |
|---|---|---|---|
| | Strip color | Level | |
| less than 0.6 | slight/no color change | negative | normal - no action needed |
| 0.6 to 1.0 | light purple | small to moderate** | extra insulin & fluids*** |
| 1.1 to 3.0 | dark purple | moderate to large** | call MD or RN** |
| greater than 3.0 | very dark purple | very large | go directly to the E.R. |

**It is usually advised to call a health care provider for a blood ketone level greater than 1.0 or with urine ketone readings of moderate or large.

***If the blood glucose level is below 150 mg/dl (8.3 mmol/L), a liquid with sugar (e.g., juice) should be taken.

# Chapter 6
# Low Blood Sugar
## (Hypoglycemia or Insulin Reaction)

Anyone who has been given insulin can have low blood sugar (hypoglycemia or a "reaction"). **A true low blood sugar is a value less than 60 mg/dl (3.3 mmol/L).**

**Main Causes:**

- 🐾 late or missed meals or snacks

- 🐾 extra exercise (the low may be "delayed" during the night)

- 🐾 too much insulin/wrong dose

- 🐾 taking bath, shower or hot tub too soon after injection (dangerous)

- 🐾 low blood sugar (for any reason, particularly at bedtime) and failing to do a follow-up blood sugar 15 to 30 minutes later, making sure the value has come up as a result of the treatment

- 🐾 illnesses, especially with vomiting

Remember that if a person has a low blood sugar and can't keep food down, low dose glucagon, one unit per year of age up to 15 units, can be given under the skin just like insulin - with an insulin syringe. The dose can be repeated every 20 minutes until the blood sugar is up. Once glucagon is mixed, it usually can continue to be used for about 24 hours before it gels.

**The signs of a low blood sugar can be different and may include:**

- 🐾 hunger

- 🐾 feeling shaky, sweaty and/or weak

- 🐾 confusion

- 🐾 sleepiness (at unusual times)

- 🐾 behavioral/mood changes

- 🐾 double vision

- 🐾 the signs of nighttime lows may be the same, or may include waking up alert, crying, or having bad dreams

Low blood sugar comes on quickly. It must be treated immediately by the person (if able) or by someone who is nearby at the time. If not treated, loss of consciousness or seizures may occur. Different levels of reactions (mild, moderate, severe) and treatment for each level are shown in the table in this chapter.

**With a "mild" low blood sugar (reaction):**
(also see table)

- give sugar (it's best in liquid form) such as four ounces of juice or sugar pop or eight ounces of milk.

- when possible, a blood sugar test should be done.

- it takes **10 to 20** minutes for the blood sugar to rise after treatment.

- re-check the blood sugar after 10 to 20 minutes to make sure the level is above 70 mg/dl (3.9 mmol/L).

- if it is still below this level, the liquid sugar should be given again. Follow the steps above, again.

- wait another 10 to 15 minutes to repeat the blood sugar test.

- if the blood sugar is above 70 mg/dl (3.9 mmol/L), give solid food. The reason for waiting to give the solid food is that it may soak up the liquid sugar and slow the time for the sugar to get into the blood.

- the person should not return to activity until the blood sugar is above 70 mg/dl (3.9 mmol/L).

- if the low is at bedtime, it is best to repeat the blood sugar test, as above, and again during the night to make sure the level stays up.

- if a low blood sugar occurs when it is time for an insulin shot, always treat the low first. Make sure the blood sugar is back up before giving the shot.

**With a "moderate" reaction:**

- put half a tube of Insta-Glucose® or cake gel between the gums and cheeks. Rub the cheeks and stroke the throat to help with swallowing.

**With a "severe" reaction:**

- if a seizure or complete loss of consciousness occurs, it may be necessary to give a shot of **glucagon**. After mixing, give the following doses under the skin (just like insulin):

  less than 5 years = 0.3 cc (30 units)

  5-16 years = 0.5 cc (50 units)

  greater than 16 years = 1.0 cc (100 units)

**Though the result of using glucagon is the opposite of insulin, it is <u>NOT</u> sugar. It will make the blood sugar rise, usually in 10 to 20 minutes.**

*Giving glucagon:*

🐾 after mixing, it can be given with an insulin syringe just like insulin.

*Amount of glucagon to give:*

🐾 under 5 can be given a full 30 unit syringe.

🐾 5-16 can be given a full 50 unit syringe.

🐾 over 16 can be given a full 100 unit syringe.

🐾 if the person does not respond in 10 to 20 minutes the paramedics (911) should be called.

Your doctor or nurse should be called prior to the next insulin shot, as the amount of insulin you give may need to be changed.

Never give a shot
and then get in a shower,
bathtub or hot tub.
The blood coming to
the skin surface may cause
the insulin to be rapidly
absorbed. This may result
in a severe insulin reaction.

# Table
# Hypoglycemia:  Treatment of Low Blood Sugar (B.S.)
### *Always check blood sugar level!*

| Low Blood Sugar Category | MILD | MODERATE | SEVERE |
|---|---|---|---|
| **Alertness** | **ALERT** | **NOT ALERT**<br><br>**Unable to drink safely (choking risk)**<br>**Needs help from another person** | **UNRESPONSIVE**<br><br>**Loss of consciousness**<br><br>**Seizure**<br><br>**Needs constant adult help (position of safety)**<br><br>*Give nothing by mouth (extreme choking risk)* |
| **Symptoms** | Mood Changes<br>Shaky, Sweaty<br>Hungry<br>Fatigue, Weak<br>Pale | Lack of Focus<br>Headache<br>Confused<br>Disoriented<br>'Out of Control' (bite, kick)<br>*Can't* Self-treat | Loss of Consciousness<br>Seizure |
| **Actions to take** | ✔ Check B.S.<br>✔ Give 2-8 oz sugary fluid (amount age dependent)<br>✔ Recheck B.S. in 10-15 min.<br>✔ B.S. < 70 mg/dl (< 3.9 mmol/L), repeat sugary fluid and recheck in 10-20 min.<br>✔ B.S. > 70 mg/dl (> 3.9 mmol/L), (give a solid snack) | ✔ *Place in position of safety*<br>✔ Check B.S.<br>✔ If on insulin pump, may disconnect or suspend until fully recovered from low blood sugar (**awake and alert**)<br>✔ Give Insta-Glucose or cake decorating gel - put between gums and cheek and rub in.<br>✔ Look for person to 'wake up'<br>✔ Recheck B.S. in 10-20 min.<br>✔ *Once alert* – follow "actions" under 'Mild' column<br><br>(Can use low dose glucagon: [1 unit per year of age], if very disoriented or out of control) | ✔ *Place in position of safety*<br>✔ Check B.S.<br>✔ If on insulin pump, disconnect or suspend until fully recovered from low blood sugar (**awake and alert**)<br>✔ Glucagon: *can be given with an insulin syringe* like insulin<br>Under 5 years : **30 units**<br>5-16 years: **50 units**<br>Over 16 years:  **100 units (all of dose)**<br>✔ If giving 50 or 100 unit doses, may use syringe in box & inject through clothing.<br>✔ **Check B.S. every 10-15 min. until > 80 mg/dl (4.5 mmol/L)**<br>✔ **If no response, may need to call 911**<br>✔ **Check B.S. every hour x 4-5 hours**<br>✔ High risk for more lows x 24 hours<br>*(need to ↑ food intake and ↓ insulin doses)* |
| **Recovery time** | 10-20 minutes | 20-45 minutes | → Call RN / MD ←<br>and report the episode<br>Effects can last 2-12 hours |

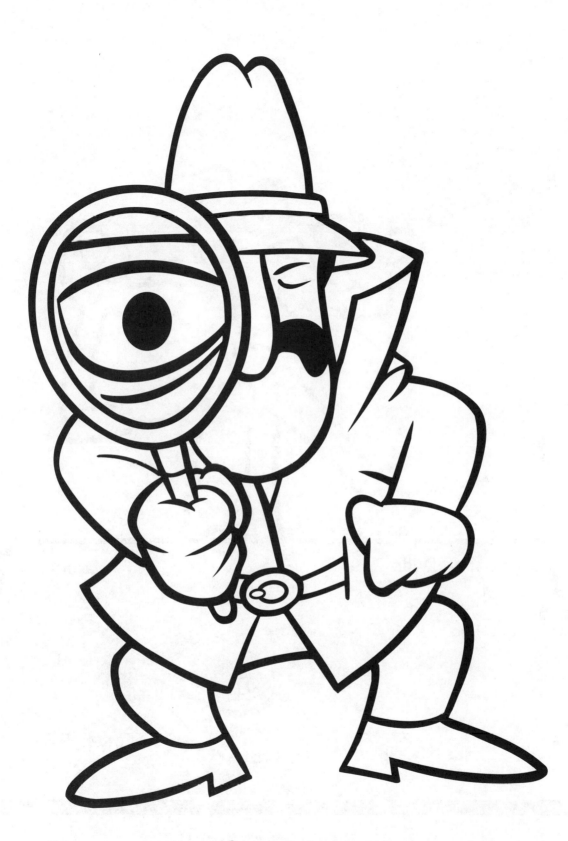

It is important for adults to keep an eye
on younger children for signs of low sugar.

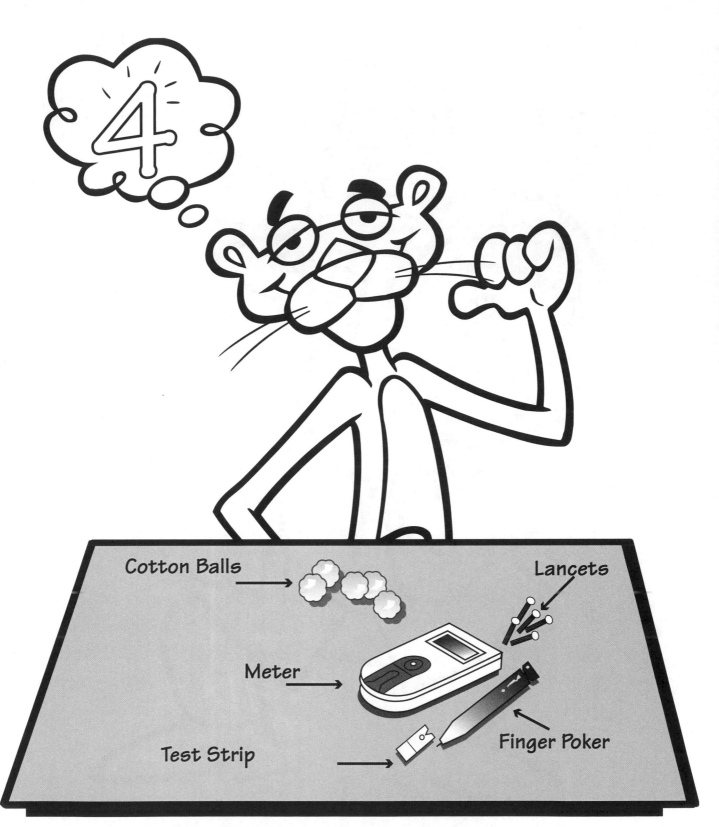

Test your blood sugars
four or more times each day.

# Chapter 7
# Blood Sugar (Glucose) Testing

## WHEN?

- four or more times each day (usually before meals and the bedtime snack)
- food should not be eaten within the two hours before a test
- at least once weekly, two hours after each meal
- anytime the symptoms of a low blood sugar are felt
- occasionally during the night
- anytime unusual symptoms occur (e.g., frequent voiding)

## Blood Sugar Level in mg/dl (mmol/L)

| | | |
|---|---|---|
| **VERY HIGH** 400-800 (22.2-44.4) | | **Stomachache Difficulty Breathing** |
| **HIGH** 200-400 (11.1-22.2) | | **Low Energy** |
| **GOALS** 80-200 (4.5-11.1) | Under 5 years | **Fine** |
| 70-180 (3.9-10.0) | 5-11 years | |
| 70-150 (3.9-8.3) | 12 years and up | |
| **LOW** below 60 (below 3.3) | True-Low | **Sweating Hunger Shakiness** |

## NON-DIABETIC NORMAL VALUES FOR CHILDREN*

| | |
|---|---|
| 70-100 (3.9-5.5) | Normal (fasting)* |
| 70-130 (3.9-7.3) | Normal (random)* |

*The DirecNet Study Group showed that approximately 95 percent of values for non-diabetic children are in this range. However, occasional values down to 60 mg/dl (3.3 mmol/L) and, for random values, up to 144 mg/dl (8.0 mmol/L) are still normal.

**ALWAYS BRING YOUR METER (and log book) TO YOUR CLINIC VISITS.**

## GOALS

The values for which to aim are different for each age group and are shown in the table below. At least half of the values at each time of day should be in the desired range for age. The values refer both to fasting and anytime food has not been eaten for two or more hours.

### Suggested Blood Sugar Levels

| Age (years) | Fasting (a.m.) or no food for 2 hours | | Bedtime (before bedtime snack or during the night) | |
| --- | --- | --- | --- | --- |
| | mg/dl | mmol/L | mg/dl | mmol/L |
| Below 5 | 80-200 | 4.5-11.1 | Above 150* [80**] | above 8.3* [4.5**] |
| 5-11 | 70-180 | 3.9-10.0 | Above 130* [70**] | above 7.3* [3.9**] |
| 12 and above | 70-150 | 3.9-8.3 | Above 130* [60**] | above 7.3* [3.3**] |

*If values are below these levels, milk or other food might be added to the solid protein and carbohydrate bedtime snack.

**If values are below these levels, the test should be rechecked 10-30 minutees later to make certain it has come back up. If this happens more than once within a week, either reduce the dinner rapid-acting or Regular insulin or call the diabetes care provider for advice.

*Note: The ADA recommended sugar levels for children of different ages vary somewhat from our suggestions. The levels for before meals and during the night recommended by the ADA can be found in Table 1 of Chapter 14.*

# DOING THE TESTING

**Finger-Pokes:** There are now many good devices. Most can be set for different depths. These may help young children or the elderly who do not need a lancet to go as deep.

**How to:**

- Get poker ready; insert lancet (change daily).

- Wash hands with soap and warm water; dry.

- Poke side or tip (not ball) of chosen finger or of arm (alternate site testing)**.

- To get enough blood, hold hand down (below heart level) and "milk" the finger.

- Wipe off the first drop of blood with a cotton ball.

- Put the second drop of blood on the test strip as taught for each meter.

- Hold cotton ball on poke site to stop bleeding.

**Meters:** We do not recommend one meter over another.

- We do like meters that can store at least the last 100 values.

- The meter must also be able to be downloaded by the family or clinic.

- Strips requiring smaller amounts of blood make it easier for young children.

- Make sure the code in the meter matches the code for the strips.

- **The meter must always be brought to the clinic visit.**

***Alternate Site Testing:*** Some meters now require such a small drop of blood that it can be obtained from the arm or another site.

**However, if feeling low, the fingertip must be used as circulation is not as good in other sites and the true blood sugar level may be delayed by 10-20 minutes.

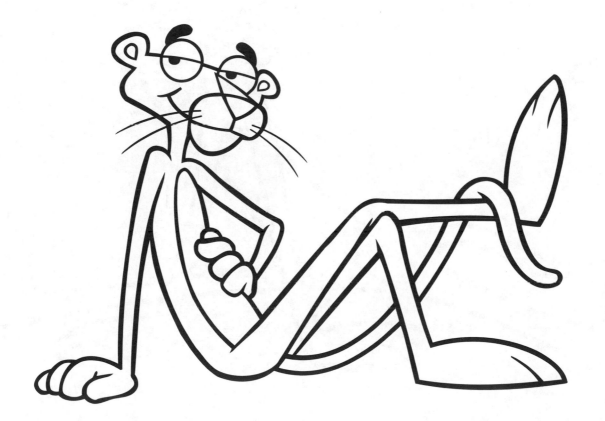

**Log books:** It is important to record results.

- Look for patterns of highs and lows.

- If too many lows occur, the results should be sent to the nurse or doctor by fax or e-mail (e.g., more than 2 values per week below 60 mg/dl [3.3 mmol/L]).

- If too many highs occur, the results should be sent to the nurse or doctor by fax or e-mail, (e.g., more than 2 values at the same time of day in a week above 300 mg/dl [16.7 mmol/L]).

- Parents (even of teens) must do or supervise the recording of the values and the sending of the results.

- **Bring the log book to the clinic visit.**

**Feelings:** It is important not to be upset if highs or lows are found. This can make testing a negative experience. Just use the data to adjust the insulin and/or to prevent future highs or lows. The only response should be **"Thank you for doing the test."**

**Continuous Glucose Monitoring (CGM)** Diabetes management is gradually moving toward CGM. This involves wearing a sensor for three to five days which will send subcutaneous (not blood) glucose values to a receiver. The CGM devices are not yet as accurate as the blood glucose meters.

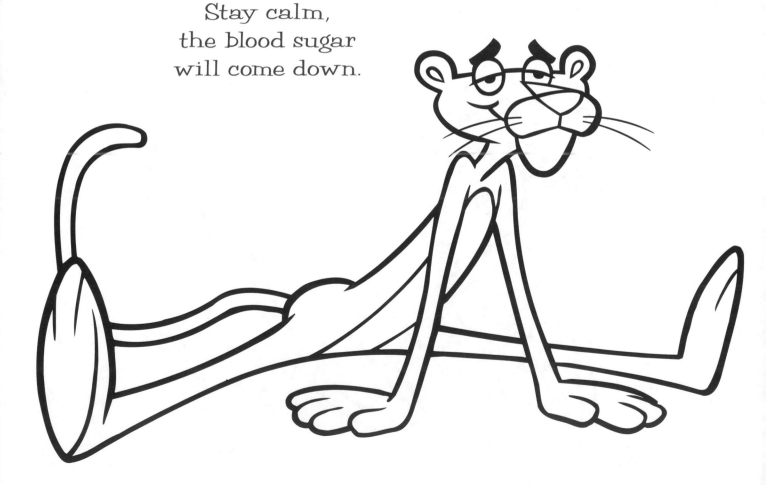

Stay calm, the blood sugar will come down.

# Chapter 8
# Insulin: Types and Activity

## WHY ARE INSULIN SHOTS NEEDED?

🐾 Not enough insulin is made in the pancreas of a person with type 1 diabetes.

🐾 Insulin can't be taken as a pill because it would be destroyed by stomach acid.

🐾 People with type 2 diabetes who have ketones or very high blood sugars also usually take insulin shots, at least in the beginning.

## THE THREE TYPES OF INSULIN ARE:

🐾① *"rapid-acting"* (Humalog, NovoLog, Apidra and Regular)

- Humalog, NovoLog and Apidra are more rapid-acting than Regular; they peak earlier and do not last as long as Regular insulin.

- Humalog, NovoLog, Apidra and Regular insulins are clear.

🐾② *"intermediate-acting"* (NPH, Lente®)

- Most intermediate-acting insulins are cloudy and must be mixed to get the same dose with each shot.

- The bottles should be turned gently up and down 20 times before drawing the insulin into the syringe.

- The NPH and Lente insulins peak during the day when food is being eaten.

🐾③ *"long-acting"* (Lantus® [insulin glargine] and Levemir® [insulin detemir]; see table)

- These are the first true basal (flat-acting, no peak) insulins that last approximately 24 hours.

- They are <u>clear</u> insulins (don't confuse with rapid-acting insulins).

- Levemir must be drawn into the syringe alone (cannot be mixed with any other insulin).

- Best given in the bottom (buttocks, seat) to make sure the insulin is given into fat or into a pinch of fat.

** *Insulin must be stored so that it does not freeze or get over 90° F (3.2° C) because it will spoil.*

# HOW AND WHEN IS INSULIN USED?

Most people take two or more shots of insulin each day.

## RAPID-ACTING INSULIN USES:

 Rapid-acting insulins are used to stop the rise of the blood sugar after eating food.

🐾 The rapid-acting insulin can be mixed with the intermediate-acting insulin to give before breakfast and dinner.

🐾 If Humalog, NovoLog or Apidra is used, it should be taken 10-15 minutes before the meal (unless the blood sugar is below 80 mg/dl [4.5 mmol/L]).

🐾 If Regular insulin is being used, the shot is usually taken 30 minutes before meals.

🐾 For toddlers: Humalog, NovoLog or Apidra can be given after the meal. That way, the dose can be adjusted to fit the amount of food eaten.

🐾 Some people also take a shot of rapid-acting insulin before lunch or the afternoon snack.

🐾 Rapid-acting insulins are also used to "correct" a blood sugar level that is too high (see Correction Insulin Dose: Chapter 21).

## Figure 1: Example of Two Injections Per Day

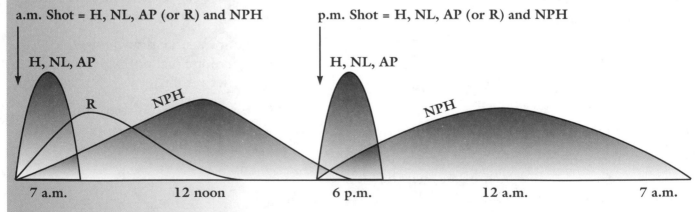

**a.m. Shot = H, NL, AP (or R) and NPH**     **p.m. Shot = H, NL, AP (or R) and NPH**

H, NL, AP     R     NPH     H, NL, AP     NPH

7 a.m.     12 noon     6 p.m.     12 a.m.     7 a.m.

Many people receive two injections per day. NPH may be used as the intermediate-acting insulin in the a.m. They can then take a rapid-acting insulin plus Lantus (see Figure 1-B) or NPH prior to dinner.

## INTERMEDIATE-ACTING INSULIN USE:

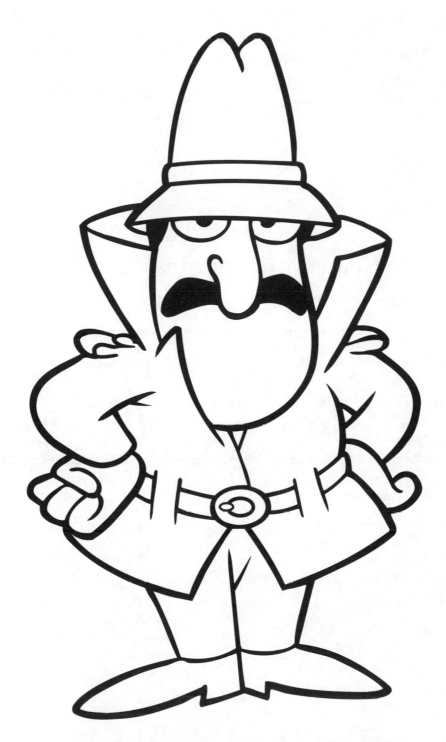

- The intermediate-acting insulins (NPH and Lente) are longer-acting peak insulins. They are usually taken twice daily in a syringe with a rapid-acting insulin.

- Intermediate-acting insulins taken at dinner or bedtime have a peak during the night so that low blood sugars are more common compared to when a basal (long-acting) insulin is used.

- People who take three shots per day sometimes take their NPH at bedtime rather than at dinner to help it last through the night.

## LONG-ACTING INSULIN USE:

🐾 When using insulin glargine (Lantus) or insulin detemir (Levemir):

- the dose is usually taken alone without any other insulin in the syringe (ask your doctor). (Then Humalog, NovoLog or Apidra are taken before each meal.) See Figure 1.

- it is best to take the insulin in the buttocks (seat) or to give the insulin into a pinch of fat in the stomach (to make sure the insulin is going into the fat).

- the action is very flat and the chance for a bad low blood sugar, particularly during the night, is reduced.

- it works as a basal insulin, which prevents the liver from releasing sugar (and ketones) into the blood.

- NPH (an intermediate-acting insulin) is sometimes taken in the morning, particularly if a noon shot cannot be taken. It can be given in the same syringe with the rapid-acting insulin. See example in Figure 1.

- the dose is judged on the basis of the morning blood sugar no matter when the Lantus or Levemir shot is taken (a.m., lunch, dinner or bedtime; all times work - though one consistent time must be chosen). If the blood sugar is consistently above the desired range (Chapter 7) at breakfast, the dose is increased. If below the lower level, the dose is decreased.

# Figure 2: Use of Lantus or Levemir Insulin

*Two of the most common methods of using Lantus or Levemir insulin:*

**Figure 1-A.** In the first example, Lantus or Levemir is used as the basal insulin (given in the a.m., or at dinner or at bedtime) and a rapid-acting insulin is taken prior to meals and snacks.

**Figure 1-B.** In this second example, NPH and a rapid-acting insulin are taken in one syringe in the a.m. A rapid-acting insulin is taken alone at dinner. Lantus or Levemir (alone in the syringe) is taken consistently either in the a.m., at dinner, or at bedtime.

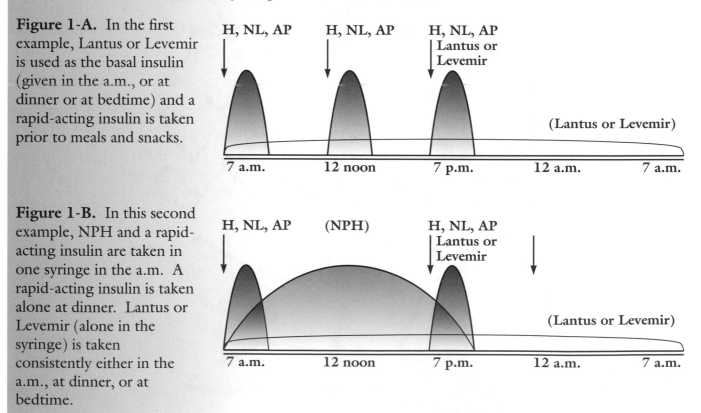

## Table 1
## Insulin Activities

| Type of Insulin | Begins Working | Main Effect | All Gone |
|---|---|---|---|
| **RAPID-ACTING and REGULAR** | | | |
| Humalog/NovoLog/Apidra | 10-15 minutes | 30-150 minutes | 5 hours |
| Regular | 30-60 minutes | 2-4 hours | 6-9 hours |
| **INTERMEDIATE-ACTING** | | | |
| NPH | 2-4 hours | 6-8 hours | 12-15 hours |
| **LONG-ACTING** | | | |
| Lantus (insulin glargine) | 1-2 hours | 2-24 hours | 24 hours |
| Levemir (insulin detemir) | 1-2 hours | 2-22 hours | 22-24 hours |
| **PRE-MIXED INSULINS** | | | |
| Lente | 1-2 hours | 6-12 hours | 15-24 hours |
| NPH/Regular (R) mix | 30-60 minutes | R = 2-4 hours<br>NPH = 6-8 hours | 12-15 hours |

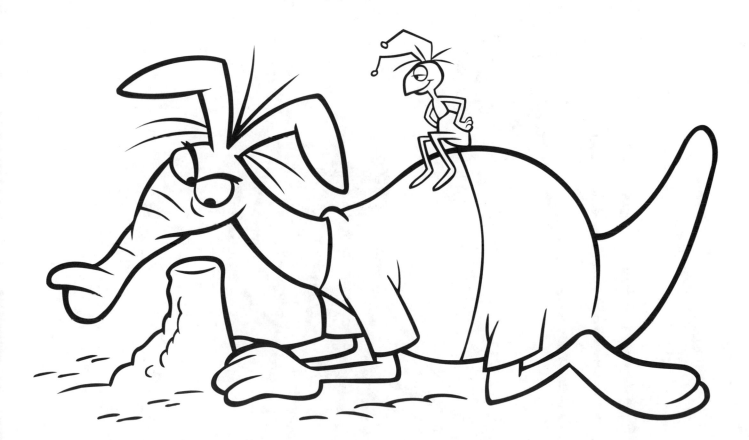

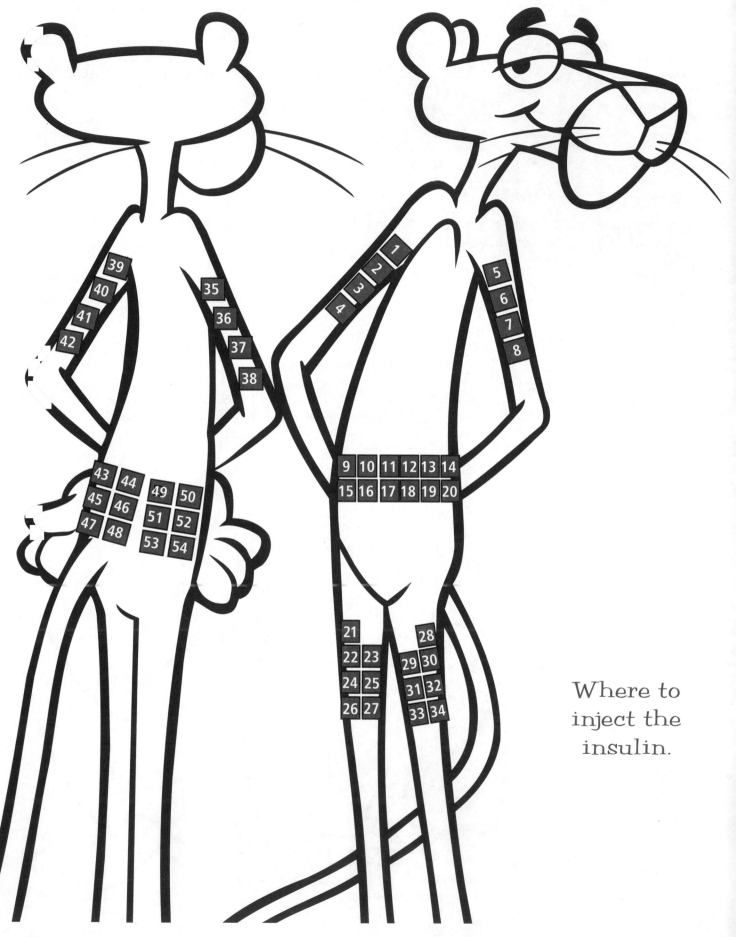

Where to inject the insulin.

# Chapter 9
# Drawing Up Insulin and Insulin Injections

The nurse-educator will teach the best way to draw up and give the insulin. Both are described below:

## DRAWING UP INSULIN

### A. <u>Get everything you will need:</u>

- a bottle of each insulin you will use

- syringe

- alcohol wipe for tops of bottles

- log book with current tests and insulin dose: please record each blood sugar result and insulin dose in log book

### B. <u>What to do:</u>

- Know how much of each insulin you need to give (based on "thinking" scales if appropriate – see Chapter 12 in <u>Understanding Diabetes</u>).

- Wipe off the tops of insulin bottles with alcohol swab.

- Inject air into the intermediate-acting (cloudy) insulin bottle with the bottle sitting upright on the table and remove the needle.*

- Inject air in the clear (rapid-acting) insulin bottle and leave the needle in the bottle.*

- Turn the rapid-acting bottle with the needle in it upside down and get rid of any air bubbles. (See this chapter for specific steps that can be used to get rid of air bubbles.) Draw up the clear rapid-acting insulin you need and remove the needle from the bottle.

- Mix the cloudy (intermediate-acting) insulin by gently turning the bottle up and down 20 times; this mixes the insulin so that it will have a consistent strength.

- Turn the bottle upside down and put the needle into the bottle. Draw up the cloudy insulin into the syringe. *Make sure not to push any rapid-acting insulin already in the syringe back into this bottle.*

- If the insulin bottles have been in the refrigerator, you can warm up the insulin once it is mixed in the syringe by holding the syringe in the closed palm of your hand for a minute. It will be less likely to sting if the insulin is at room temperature.

*An option now used by some people is to not put air into the insulin bottles, but to just "vent" the bottles once a week to remove any vacuum. This is done by removing the plunger from the syringe and inserting the needle into the upright insulin bottle. Air will be sucked in through the needle removing the vacuum from the bottle. (The vacuum may otherwise pull insulin from the syringe into the insulin bottle. This is most important if two insulins are being mixed in the same syringe.)

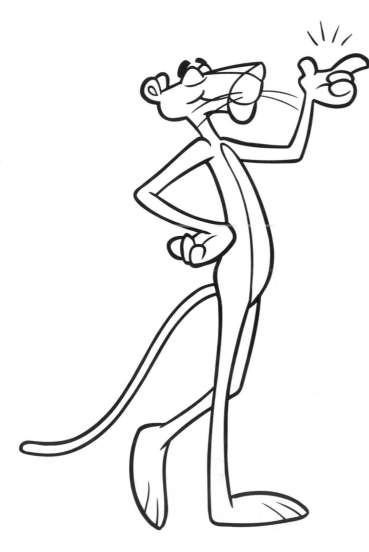

# GIVING THE INSULIN

- Choose the area of the body where you are going to give the shot. Use two or more areas and use different sites within the area.

- Make sure the area where you will be giving the shot is clean.

- Relax the chosen area.

- Pull up the skin with the finger and thumb (even with short needles).

- Touch the needle to the skin and "punch" it through the skin.

**Short Needle**
- a 90° angle for the 5/16 inch (short) needle: (these hurt less and are not as likely to go into muscle) (a 90° angle looks like this: _____ )

**Long Needle**
- use a 45° angle for the 5/8 inch needle (only) (a 45° angle looks like this: _____ )

- Push in the insulin slowly and steadily; wait five to 10 seconds to let the insulin spread out.

- Let go of the skin pulled up.

- Put a finger or dry cotton over the needle as it is pulled out; gently rub a few times to close the hole where the needle was inserted; press your finger or the cotton down on the area where you gave the shot if bruising or bleeding happens.

- Look to see if a drop of insulin comes back through the hole the needle made ("leak-back"); make a note in your log book if this happens.

The nurse will teach the right way to give shots so that a drop of insulin does not leak-back. A drop can contain as much as five units of insulin.

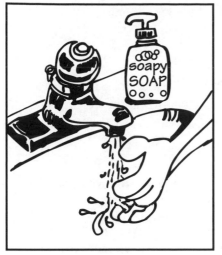

A. Wash hands

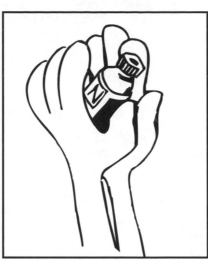

B. Warm and mix insulin

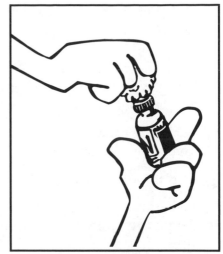

C. Wipe top of insulin bottle with alcohol

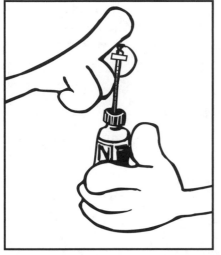

D. Air = insulin dose in units

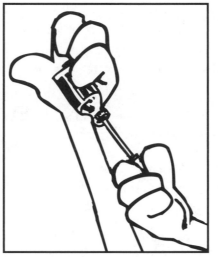

E. Pull out dose of insulin

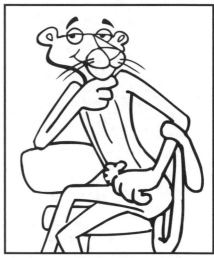

F. Make sure injection site is clean

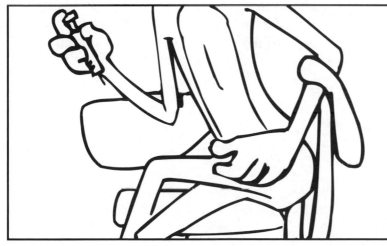

G. Pinch up skin and fat tissue.
If using 5/8 inch needle, go in at angle.
If using the 5/16 inch (short) needle, can go straight in.

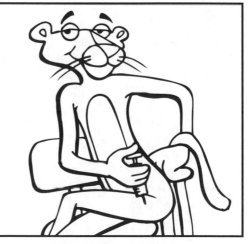

H. Basal insulins (Lantus, Levemir) are best given in the buttock.

# CHILDREN AND INSULIN SHOTS

 A young child can help with choosing where the shot will be given and by holding still.

 Children usually begin to give some of their own shots around age 10.

 It is important that both mom and dad share in giving shots.

 Some age-related issues (see Chapter 18) are:

### Toddlers:

• This age group can sometimes fight when having to get shots. The Inject-Ease® is a device that helps some families.

• Some toddlers are helped by the Insuflon® (see this chapter).

• Keep the area where the shot will be given as still as possible. Try to get the child's attention on something else (e.g., television, blowing bubbles, looking at a book, etc.). This will help the child to relax.

• The buttocks are often used first, and later the legs and arms and tummy.

• With the child's permission, the Lantus or Levemir insulin can be given when the child is asleep.

• The parent must remember when giving their child a shot they are giving them health.

### School age:

• The child may help in choosing the area on their body to give the shot.

• Change where the shots are given. Use two or more areas and use different sites within the area.

### Teens:

• Many teens give their own shots and do not want help.

• It is still important to give the shots in a place (e.g., the kitchen) where parents can actually see the shot given.

• Parents can stay involved by helping to get the supplies out, and helping to keep records by writing down the blood sugars and insulin doses each day (in the log book).

## INSUFLON

The Insuflon is a small plastic cannula that can be placed under the skin (using EMLA cream to reduce pain, if desired) for giving all insulin shots. It is much like the cannula for an insulin pump (Chapter 26) but instead has a port for injecting the insulin. Twisting the syringe (or pen) helps to get the needle in. Some families inject two units of saline before or after Lantus. Glucagon (e.g., at school) can also be given into the Insuflon. It can be left in for three to five days. It can be obtained from Liberty at 1-800-467-8546.

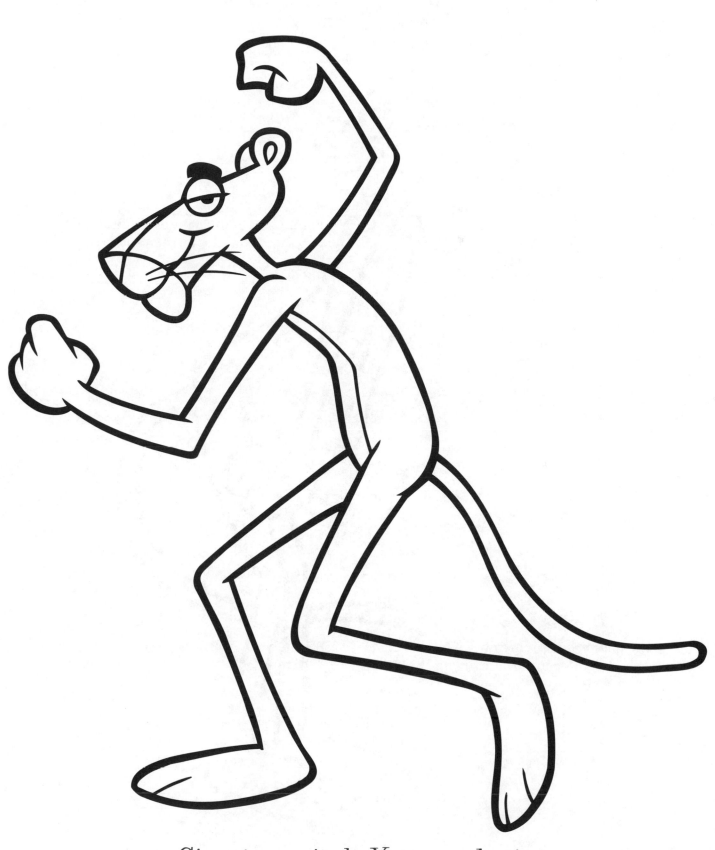

Stay in control. You can do it.

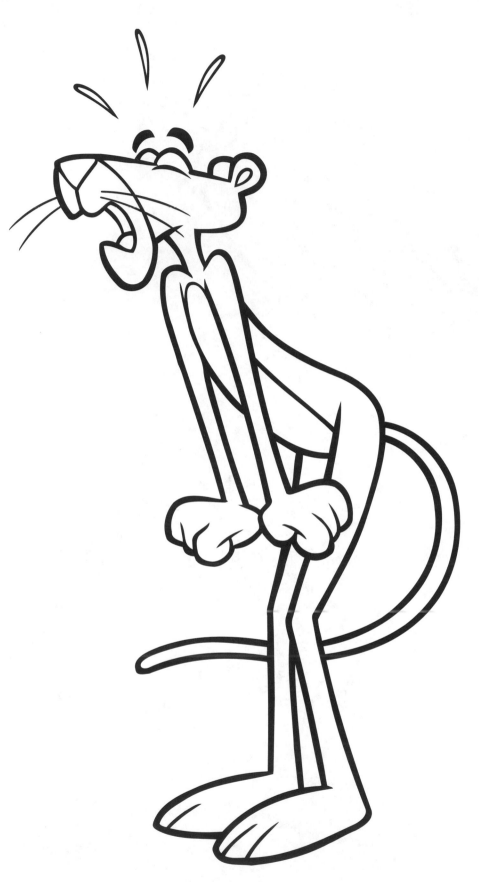

Anger, shock, and denial are common feelings
when you first learn you have diabetes.

# Chapter 10
# Feelings and Diabetes

You and your child will have many feelings when you find out about the diabetes. Having these feelings is very normal. It is important for families to share and talk about these feelings.

The most common feelings are:

- **shock**
- **grief**
- **denial**
- **sadness**
- **anger**
- **fear/anxiety**
- **guilt**
- **adapting: as time passes, everyone will not feel so overwhelmed**

We ask **EVERY** newly diagnosed family to meet with a counselor to discuss feelings. It is important for all family members to share how they feel. All family members need to work toward feeling positive about how diabetes will fit into their family life.

As time passes, the family will find they are better able to deal with the shots, blood sugar checks, food plan and other day to day tasks. More talking within the family and with their health care givers can help reduce the stress.

Fitting the diabetes into as normal a lifestyle as possible becomes the major goal.

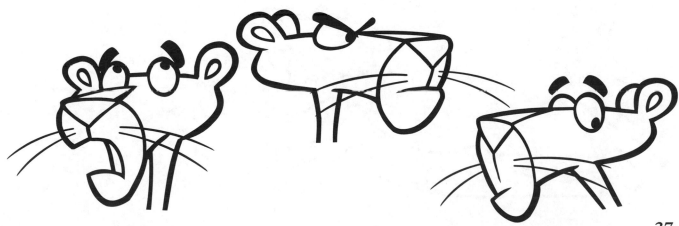

# The Healthy Eating Pyramid

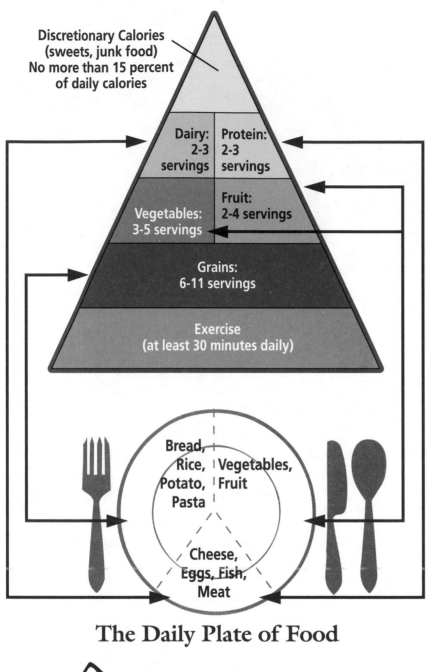

**Discretionary Calories (sweets, junk food)**
No more than 15 percent of daily calories

Dairy: 2-3 servings | Protein: 2-3 servings

Fruit: 2-4 servings

Vegetables: 3-5 servings

Grains: 6-11 servings

Exercise (at least 30 minutes daily)

Bread, Rice, Potato, Pasta | Vegetables, Fruit

Cheese, Eggs, Fish, Meat

## The Daily Plate of Food

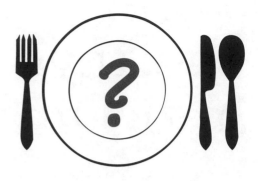

**What does your plate for a day look like?**

**Look at the food guide to see if you need to:**

- Eat more starch foods (e.g., whole wheat bread, brown rice, potato and pasta)

- Eat more fruits and vegetables

- Eat less protein and fat (particularly red meat)

- In general eat more foods that are low on the pyramid and fewer foods that are higher

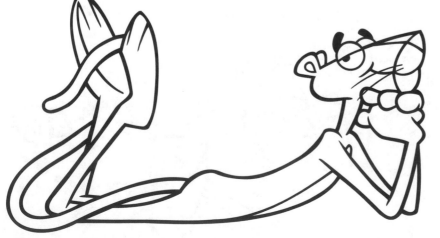

The food pyramid — Try to eat more of the foods in the lower three blocks.

# Chapter 11
# Normal Nutrition

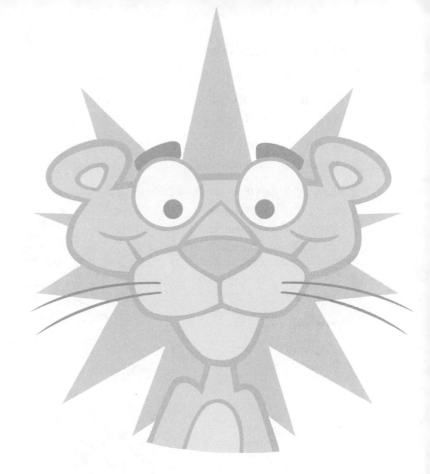

Some knowledge of normal nutrition helps when working with the dietitian on a diabetes food plan.

The foods we eat are divided into:

- **proteins**
- **carbohydrates (includes all sugars)**
- **fats**
- **vitamins and minerals**
- **water**
- **fiber**

All of these are important for our bodies and are discussed in more detail in *"Understanding Diabetes."*

Insulin has its main effect on sugars. It is important to eat high-sugar foods only when there is enough insulin acting in the body.

It used to be thought that simple sugars (e.g., candy) were quickly absorbed in the stomach and complex sugars (e.g., starch) were slowly absorbed. This is now known

**NOT** to be true. All carbohydrates are used at the same rate so they increase blood sugars in the same way.

Remember, **"a carbohydrate is a carbohydrate is a carbohydrate..."**

**It is more important to think about the following:**

🐾 **WHEN** carbohydrate is eaten. (Do not constantly snack between meals, or else blood sugars will be high.)

🐾 **HOW MUCH** carbohydrate is eaten. (A can of sugar pop has 10 teaspoons of sugar and is a "load" for anyone.)

🐾 **WITH WHAT** the carbohydrate is eaten. (Other foods, such as fat, slow the sugar absorption.)

🐾 **IF INSULIN IS ACTING** at the same time the sugar is eaten, which allows the carbohydrate to pass into cells for energy (see Chapter 2).

Other thoughts discussed in Chapter 11 of _Understanding Diabetes_ are:

- Working with the dietitian helps families keep up-to-date on new dietary ideas.

- Learning to read nutrition labels on foods at the store is very important.

- Having a normal level of blood fats (e.g., cholesterol) is important for people with diabetes. These levels can be tested once yearly at a clinic visit.

Eating nutritious foods will help all family members.

# Chapter 12
# Food Management and Diabetes

A food plan is important for people with either type 1 or type 2 diabetes. Every family must work out a plan with their dietitian that fits their family.

Type 1 diabetes <u>cannot</u> be treated with diet alone.

*People with type 2 diabetes:*

🐾 can sometimes be treated with diet and exercise alone

🐾 need to eat foods with fewer calories each day and lose weight

- must reduce fat calories (fat has nine calories per gram; carbohydrate [carbs] and protein have four calories per gram)

- should not eat more than once a week at fast food restaurants (burger, fries, pizza)

*The two types of food plans that our clinic uses the most are:*

🐾① **Constant carbohydrate:** A family often starts with this plan.

- This plan involves eating about the same amount of carbs for each meal and for each snack from day to day.

- Insulin doses are changed based on the blood sugar level ("sliding scale"), exercise, and other factors such as illness, stress, menses, etc. ("thinking scale").

🐾② **Carbohydrate ("carb") counting:** Families often move to this plan at a later date.

- This plan involves counting the grams of carbohydrate (carbs) in food to be eaten. An amount of rapid-acting insulin is given that matches the number of grams (g) of carbohydrate (I/C ratio = insulin to carb ratio).

- The healthcare team and family choose an insulin-to-carb ratio (I/C ratio).

- The dietitian may want a three-day diet record to be done first.

- The ratio which is often used when starting this plan is one unit of insulin for each 15g of carbohydrate (I/C ratio of 1 to 15).

- Blood sugars are then done 2 hours after meals to see if the I/C ratio is correct.

  If the blood sugar level is high (e.g., over 180 mg/dl or 10.0 mmol/L), the ratio could be changed to one unit of insulin for 10g of carbs (I/C ratio of 1 to 10).

  If the blood sugar level is low (e.g., less than 60 mg/dl or 3.3 mmol/L), the ratio could be changed to one unit of insulin for 20g of carbs (I/C ratio of 1 to 20).

- Gradually the correct ratios for each meal are found. The I/C ratio may vary between meals.

- A blood sugar is done and an insulin dose "correction factor" (see Chapter 21) is usually added to the I/C ratio dose. This will be the total dose of insulin to be given before the meal or snack.

- If blood sugars are above the desired upper level one or two hours after meals (and the pre-meal blood sugar is above 90 mg/dl [5.0 mmol/L], it may be helpful to give the pre-meal rapid-acting insulin 15 to 30 minutes before meals. This is because blood sugar levels peak in 60 minutes after a meal, whereas Humalog/NovoLog/Apidra insulins do not peak until 100 minutes.

Several tables of the carb contents of foods and more details about carb counting are found in Chapter 12 of *Understanding Diabetes*.

**Some beginning rules of good food management, some of which relate more to a constant carb food plan, are:**

- eat a well-balanced diet

- keep the diet similar from day to day

- eat meals and snacks at the same time each day

- use snacks to prevent insulin reactions (see suggested snacks in Chapter 12 of *Understanding Diabetes*)

- carefully watch how much carbohydrate is eaten

- avoid over-treating low blood sugars

- eat foods with less cholesterol and saturated fats; reduce total fat intake

- keep appropriate growth

- watch weight for height; avoid becoming overweight

- increase the amount of fiber eaten

- eat fewer foods that are high in salt (sodium)

- avoid eating too much protein

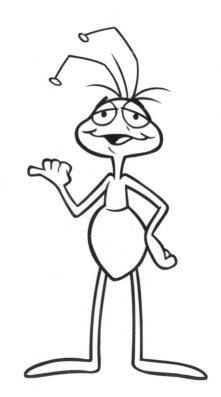

A study known as the **DCCT\*** found six dietary factors that made sugar control better:

 1. following some sort of a meal plan

2. not eating extra snacks

3. not over-treating low blood sugars (hypoglycemia)

4. prompt treatment of high blood sugars when found

5. adjusting insulin levels for meals

 6. consistency of bedtime snacks

As shown in the diagram in Chapter 14, food is one of the four major influences on blood sugar control.

**\*DCCT:** Diabetes Control and Complications Trial (see Chapter 14).

Make sure you eat a bedtime snack that has solid protein, fat and carbohydrate

(especially if a heavy exercise day, if the blood sugar is below 130 mg/dl [7.3 mmol/L] or if a peak [NPH, Lente] insulin is taken at night).

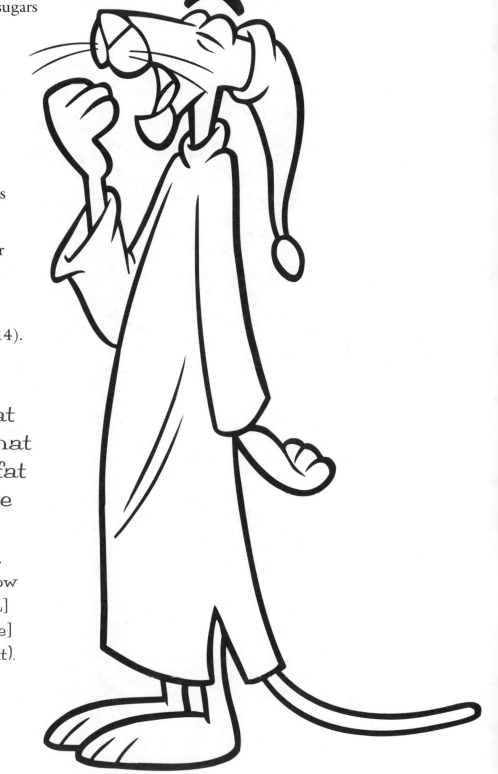

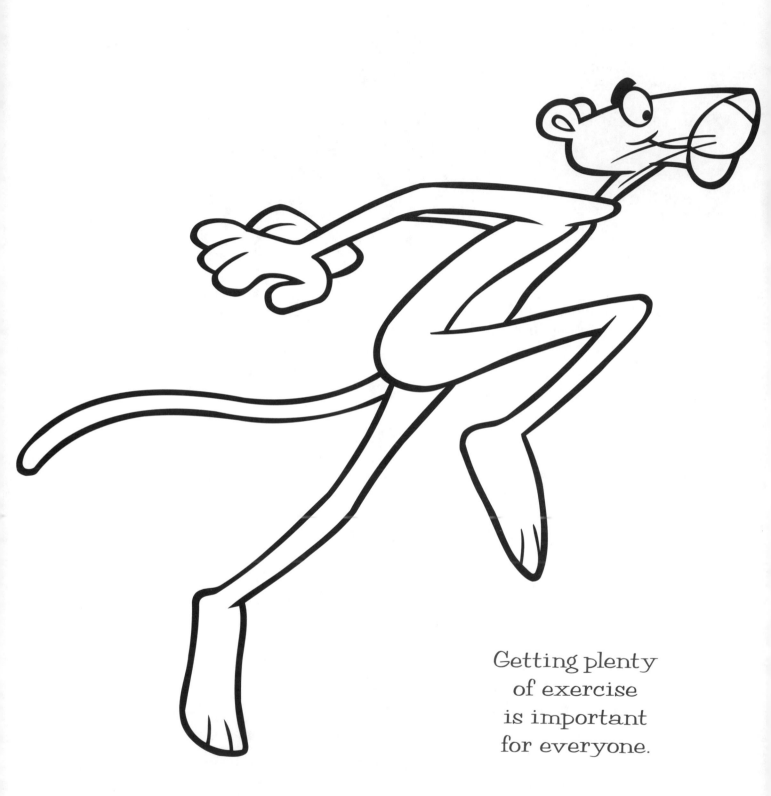

Getting plenty
of exercise
is important
for everyone.

# Chapter 13
# Exercise and Diabetes

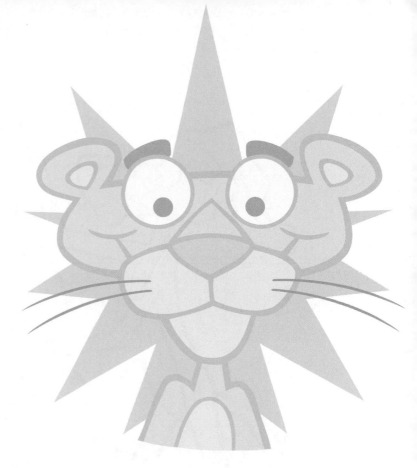

Regular exercise is important for everyone. It may be more important for people with diabetes. For people with type 2 diabetes, regular exercise and eating less food are two of the most important parts of treating the diabetes (see Chapter 4).

## Blood Sugars With and Without One Hour of Exercise

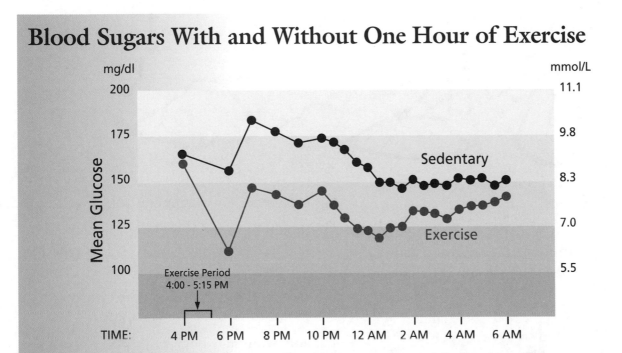

This Figure presents blood glucose (sugar) levels for the same 50 children on a sedentary day (black circles) and an exercise day (red circles). The one hour of exercise at 4 p.m. resulted in lower glucose levels for the next 14 hours (through the night). Insulin doses and food intake were identical for the two days.

*(Data complements of the DirecNet Study Group: J Pediatr 147,528, 2005)*

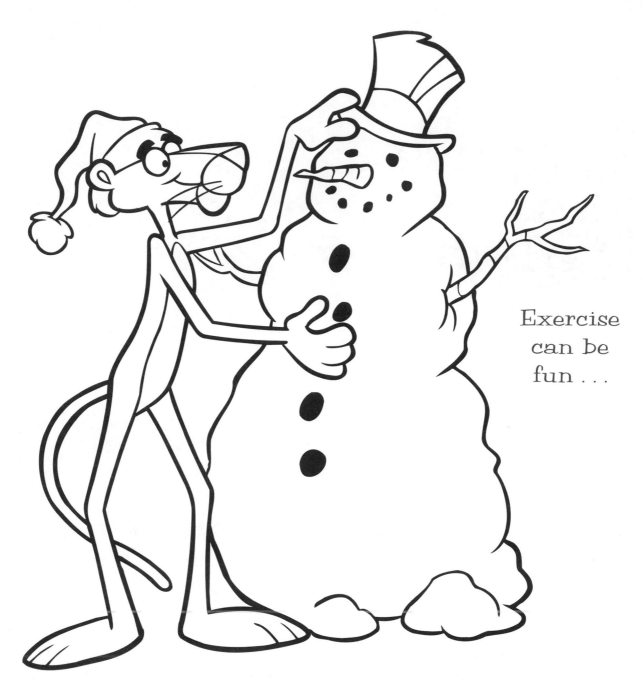

Exercise
can be
fun . . .

# EXERCISE:

🐾 is one of the "big four," which, along with insulin or oral medicines, food and stress affects blood sugar levels (see figure in Chapter 14).

🐾 may lower or raise (due to adrenaline output ) the blood sugar level. Over-all it helps to keep the blood sugars in a good range. It does this in part by making us more sensitive to insulin.

🐾 is a primary part of treating type 2 diabetes.

🐾 is essential for weight control.

🐾 should be done daily for at least 30 minutes by people with type 1 or type 2 diabetes.

🐾 can cause **low blood sugars** (Chapter 6) so it is important to plan ahead.

The following may help:

• Extra snacks or less insulin may be needed.

• Aiming for a higher blood sugar level before exercise (e.g., 180 mg/dl [10.0 mmol/L]).

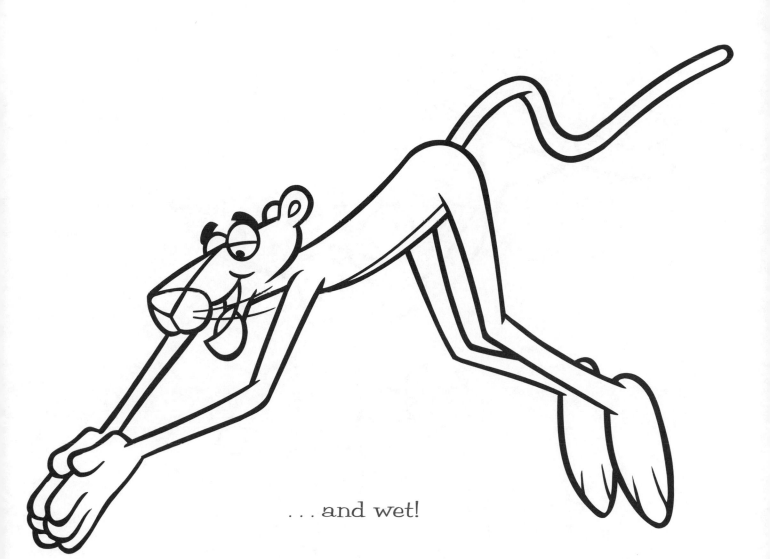

. . . and wet!

- Thinking ahead to prevent low blood
  sugars during or up to 12 hours after
  ("delayed hypoglycemia") the exercise.
  - ~ The evening insulin dose may need to
    be reduced.
  - ~ Adding an extra 15 or 30 grams of
    carbohydrate at bedtime if afternoon
    or evening exercise has been
    strenuous.
  - ~ Making sure the bedtime blood sugar
    is above 130 mg/dl (7.3 mmol/L)
- Use of drinks such as Gatorade® during
  hard exercise.

- Doing extra blood sugar tests can be very
  helpful.
- Drinking extra water during exercise
  prevents dehydration.
- Regular exercise may also be important
  for people with diabetes in helping to
  keep normal foot circulation in later
  years.

Learn to balance
food, insulin
(or oral medicines),
stress, and exercise
for good sugar
control.

## Chapter 14
# Diabetes and Blood Sugar Control

People with diabetes whose blood sugars are mostly in the desired range for age are said to be in "good sugar control" (blood sugar is the same thing as blood glucose). Goals for blood sugars are given in this chapter and Chapter 7.

## SUGAR CONTROL:

🐾 is measured day to day by checking blood sugar levels on a meter (or, more recently, by a continuous glucose monitor [CGM]).

🐾 is also measured by a very important test called the hemoglobin $A_{1c}$ test (**$HbA_{1c}$ or $A_{1c}$**).

**The HbA1c test:**

- can be thought of as the **"forest"** and the blood sugars as the **"trees"**

- tells how often the sugars have been high for every second of the day for the past 90 days

- should be done every three months

- should be in the desired range (see table) for a person to be in "good sugar control."

## WHY IS GOOD SUGAR CONTROL IMPORTANT?

**Good Sugar Control (lower HbA1c values):**

 helps people feel better.

 can lessen the risk for the eye, kidney, nerve and heart problems from diabetes. This was proven by The **DCCT** (**D**iabetes **C**ontrol and **C**omplications **T**rial).

 helps to lower blood fats (cholesterol and triglyceride levels; see Chapter 11).

 helps children grow to their full adult height.

49

# Normal Ranges and Goals for HbA$_{1c}$ and Blood Sugar Values

| | HbA$_{1c}$* | Blood Sugar** |
|---|---|---|
| Normal values (non-diabetic): | 4.3-6.2% | 70-120 (3.9-6.7) |
| **Goals for someone with diabetes:** | | |
| 19 years or older | less than 7% | 70-140 (3.9-7.8) |
| 13-19 years | less than 7.5% | 70-150 (3.9-8.3) |
| 6-12 years | less than 8% | 70-180 (3.9-10.0) |
| under six years old | 7.5%-8.5% | 80-200 (4.5-11.1) |

*Some care providers are now suggesting all children should aim for an HbA$_{1c}$ below 8%, and adults should aim for a level below 7%.

**Blood sugar values are given in mg/dl with the mmol/L in parentheses. These levels should be the goal for both fasting (e.g., AM) and two hours after meals.

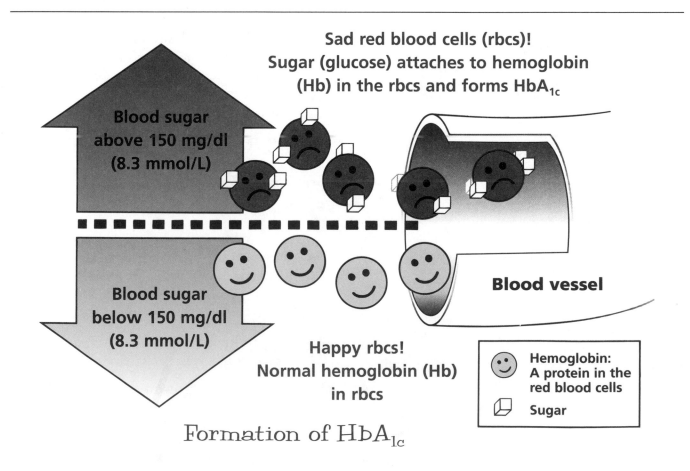

Formation of HbA$_{1c}$

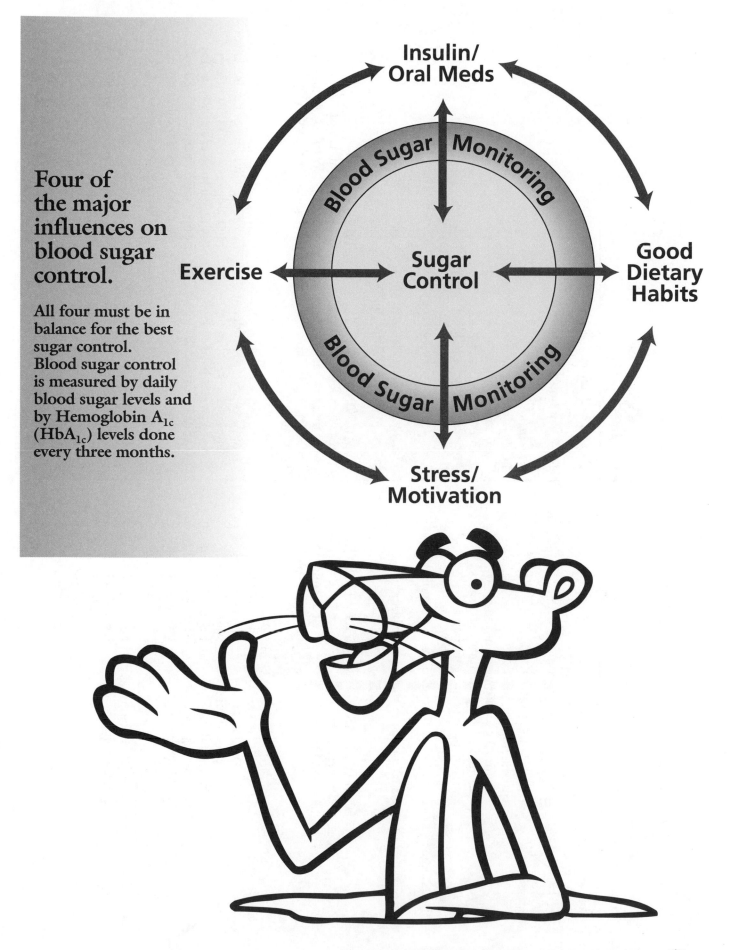

**Four of the major influences on blood sugar control.**

All four must be in balance for the best sugar control. Blood sugar control is measured by daily blood sugar levels and by Hemoglobin $A_{1c}$ (Hb$A_{1c}$) levels done every three months.

Insulin/
Oral Meds

Blood Sugar Monitoring

Exercise

Sugar Control

Good Dietary Habits

Blood Sugar Monitoring

Stress/
Motivation

## Table
## The Two Emergencies of Diabetes

| | Low Blood Sugar (Chapter 6) (Hypoglycemia or Insulin Reaction) | Ketoacidosis (Chapter 15) (Acidosis or DKA) |
|---|---|---|
| Due to: | Low blood sugar | Presence of ketones |
| Time of onset: | Fast – within seconds | Slow – in hours or days |
| Causes: | Too little food<br>Too much insulin<br>Too much exercise without food<br>Missing or being late for meals/snacks<br>Excitement in young children | Too little insulin<br>Not giving insulin<br>Infections/Illness<br>Traumatic body stress<br>Pump insertions malfunctioning |
| Blood sugar: | Low (below 60 mg/dl or 3.3 mmol/L) | Usually high (over 240 mg/dl or 13.3 mmol/L) |
| Ketones: | Usually none in the urine or blood | Usually moderate/large in the urine or blood ketones over 0.6 mmol/L. |
| | **SYMPTOMS** | **SYMPTOMS** |
| Mild: | Hunger, shaky, sweaty, nervous | Thirst, frequent urination, sweet breath, small or moderate urine ketones or blood ketones less than 1.0 mmol/L. |
| Moderate: | Headache, unexpected behavior changes, impaired or double vision, confusion, drowsiness, weakness or difficulty talking. | Dry mouth, nausea, stomach cramps, vomiting, moderate or large urine ketones or blood ketones between 1.0 and 3.0 mmol/L. |
| Severe: | Loss of consciousness or seizures. | Labored deep breathing, extreme weakness, confusion and eventually unconsciousness (coma): large urine ketones or blood ketones above 3.0 mmol/L. |
| | **TREATMENT** | **TREATMENT** |
| Mild: | Give juice or milk. Wait 10 minutes and then give solid food. | Give lots of fluids and Humalog/NovoLog/Apidra **or** Regular insulin every two or three hours. |
| Moderate: | Give instant glucose or a fast-acting sugar, juice or sugar pop (4 oz). After 10 minutes, give solid food. | Continued contact with healthcare provider. Give lots of fluids. Give Humalog/NovoLog/Apidra or Regular insulin every two or three hours. Give Phenergan medication (suppository or topical cream) if vomiting occurs. |
| Severe: | Give glucagon into muscle or fat. Test blood sugar. If no response, call paramedic (911) or go to E.R. | ***Go to the emergency room.*** May need intravenous fluids and insulin. |

# Chapter 15
# Ketonuria and Acidosis
## (Diabetic Ketoacidosis or DKA)

This is the second emergency (the other being low blood sugar) of type 1 diabetes.

## WHAT LEADS TO DKA?

DKA occurs when *ketones* build up in the body because there isn't enough insulin.

*Ketones* are:

- made by the body from breaking down fat when sugar cannot be used for energy (not enough insulin in the body)

- an acid that forms when the body uses fat for the energy it needs

## HOW DOES IT START?

- The body will first spill ketones in the urine (**ketonuria**) when there isn't enough insulin.

- If the body still doesn't get the insulin it needs, then the ketone (acid) level in the blood builds up (**DKA: D**iabetic **K**eto**A**cidosis).

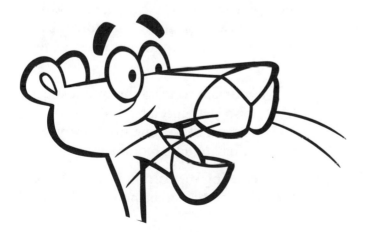

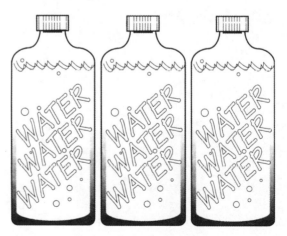

High blood sugar will make you thirsty. Drinking fluids helps "wash-out" ketones.

## WHAT ARE THE MAIN CAUSES OF KETONURIA OR OF DKA?

 Forgetting to give one or more insulin shots. Giving "spoiled" insulin (insulin that got too hot [over 90° F, 32° C] or froze).

 Illness: the amount of insulin needed is usually more so the body will have the extra energy it needs to fight the illness.

 Not enough insulin (dose too small).

An insulin pump that is not working or has been disconnected from the body.

Traumatic stress on the body (particularly type 2 diabetes).

DKA can be very dangerous. It usually does not occur unless large urine ketones or blood ketones above 3.0 mmol/L have been present for several hours. It usually occurs in people with known diabetes who forget to check blood or urine ketones as instructed (see below).

## WHAT SHOULD BE DONE TO PREVENT DKA?

- check for blood or urine ketones:

  - any time the morning blood sugar is above 240 mg/dl (13.3 mmol/L)

  - any time the blood sugar is above 300 mg/dl (16.7 mmol/L) at any time of day

  - with any illness (**even vomiting one time**)

- Call the diabetes care provider immediately if urine ketones are found to be moderate or large or if the blood ketones are above 1.0 mmol/L.

- When moderate or large urine ketones or blood ketones above 1.0 mmol/L are found, extra rapid-acting insulin is given every two to three hours to help stop ketones from being made.

- The family should then make repeat calls every two to three hours to the doctor or nurse. Extra doses of rapid-acting insulin will be needed every two hours until the high blood ketones or the moderate or large urine ketones are gone.

- It is also important to drink extra liquids. The extra liquids help to wash out the ketones.

- It is best **NOT** to exercise as the ketone level may increase. When the blood sugar is below 150 mg/dl (8.3 mmol/L), juices and other liquids with sugar can be added.

- It is important to keep the blood sugar level up so that enough insulin can be given to turn off ketone production without having low blood sugar.

- People taking metformin (Glucophage) should stop this medicine until the illness is over.

We have found that DKA can be prevented 95% of the time if the instructions in this chapter are followed.

## WHAT ARE THE SIGNS OF DKA?

- Usually the blood sugar is high. High blood sugars cause thirst and frequent urination.

- A stomachache, vomiting, or a sweet odor to the breath can occur with high ketones.

- Large urine ketones or blood ketones above 3.0 mmol/L have been present for many hours, deep or troubled breathing can occur. This is a sign to go to the emergency room.

High blood sugar will make you go the bathroom more often.

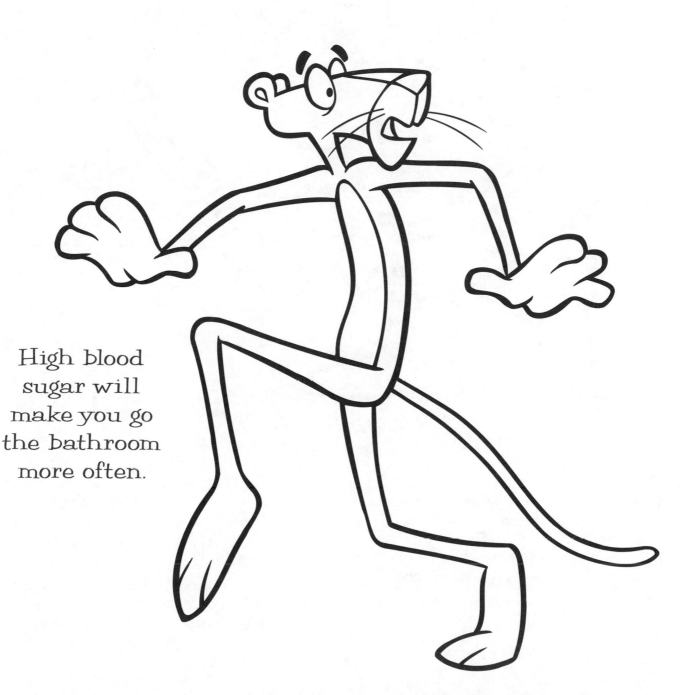

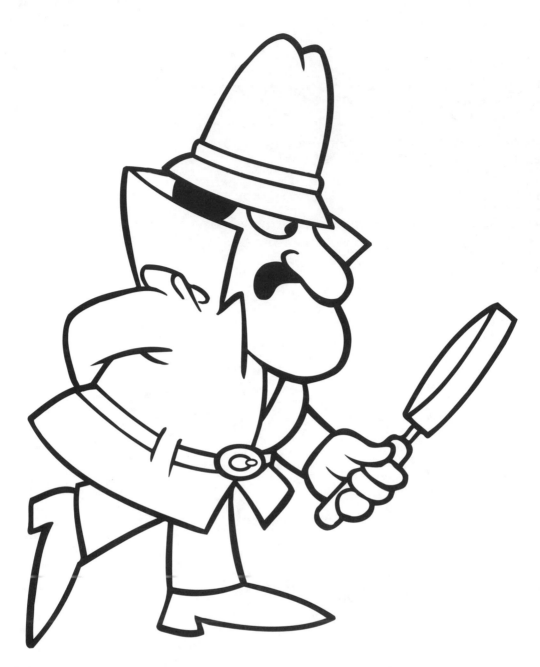

## HOW TO CHECK FOR KETONES:

*<u>*Blood sample:*</u> the most important ketone (called beta-hydroxybutyrate [ß-OHB]) can be measured with the Precision Xtra™ meter. The blood ketone test result is given as a number and is the most accurate method to use.

<u>*Urine sample:*</u> check a urine sample using a urine dipstick test such as Ketostix™ that measures a different ketone (called acetoacetic acid). Then compare the color of the pad on the stick with the color chart. The test result is read as negative, trace, small, moderate, large or very large.

*One research study found that families were more likely to test for ketones with illness if they used the <u>**blood/meter**</u> (91%) as compared with those using a urine dipstick (56%).

## Table
## Comparison of Blood and Urine Ketone Readings

| Blood Ketone (mmol/L) | Urine Ketone | | Action to take |
| --- | --- | --- | --- |
| | Strip color | Level | |
| less than 0.6 | slight/no color change | negative | normal - no action needed |
| 0.6 to 1.0 | light purple | small to moderate** | extra insulin & fluids*** |
| 1.1 to 3.0 | dark purple | moderate to large** | call MD or RN** |
| greater than 3.0 | very dark purple | very large | go directly to the E.R. |

**It is usually advised to call a health care provider for a blood ketone level greater than 1.0 or with urine ketone readings of moderate or large.

***If the blood glucose level is below 150 mg/dl (8.3 mmol/L), a liquid with sugar (e.g., juice) should be taken.

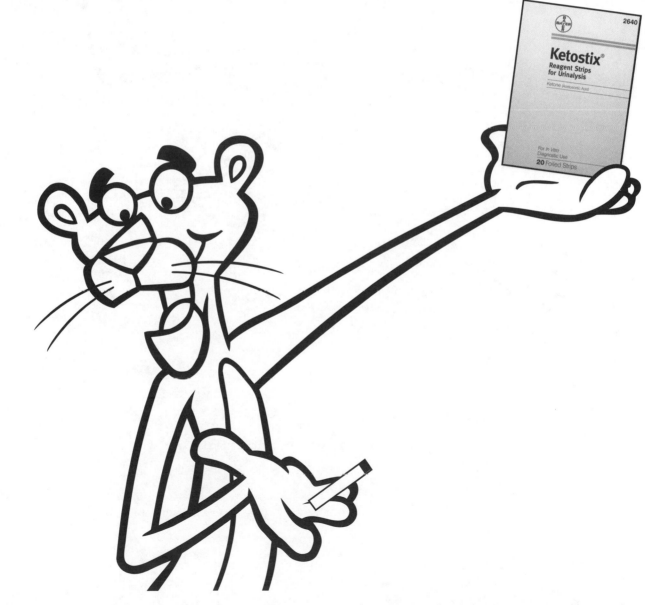

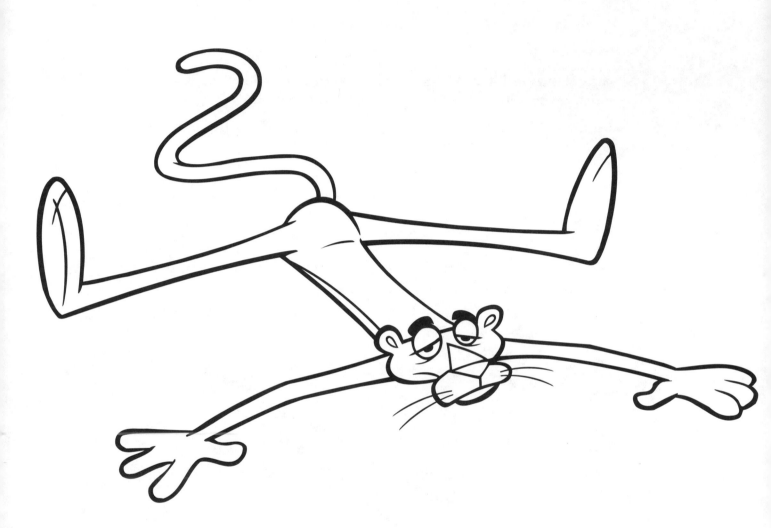

Check your ketones before calling your doctor
when you aren't feeling well.

# Chapter 16
# Sick-Day and Surgery Management

## SICK-DAY MANAGEMENT

Children with diabetes get sick just like other children. The average child gets eight colds a year. These may affect the diabetes.

It is important to:

 Always check **urine and/or blood ketones** and the **blood sugar** with any illness. Check ketones even if the blood sugar is normal.

- Call your doctor or nurse if the urine ketone result is moderate or large or if the blood ketone level (using the Precision Xtra™ meter) is above 1.0 mmol/L.

- The earlier you treat the ketones with extra Humalog/NovoLog/Apidra or Regular insulin and fluids, the less chance your child will have to go into the hospital.

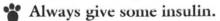 **Always give some insulin.**

- If vomiting is present and ketones are negative, the dose may have to be lowered, but some insulin **must** be given.

- If the person vomits three or more times, a Phenergan suppository or skin-application or orally dissolved tablets called Zofran® may be helpful (children under two years of age should not use a Phenergan suppository).

 Glucagon can be mixed and given with an insulin syringe just like insulin.

- It is helpful when the blood sugar is low and vomiting continues (see Chapter 6).

- The dose is one unit for every year of age up to 15 units.

- It should <u>not</u> be given if urine ketones are moderate or large (or blood ketones above 1.0 mmol/L).

- Call your doctor or nurse before giving the glucagon injection if you have questions. It can be repeated every 20 minutes if needed.

- Many medications have a warning label that a person with diabetes should not use the medicine. This is because they may raise the blood sugar a few points.

  - Our view is that if the medicine is needed, go ahead and take it. We can always give a bit more insulin if needed.

  - Steroids (e.g., prednisone) are the most difficult (often used for asthma) and, if prescribed, the diabetes care provider should be notified.

- Youth with type 2 diabetes must also remember to check the urine and/or blood ketone level.

  - If the person is receiving metformin (Glucophage), the pills should be stopped during the illness. (A condition called lactic acidosis can develop.)

  - It is usually best to return to insulin shots during the illness.

  - Call your doctor or nurse if you have questions.

# SURGERY MANAGEMENT

If surgery is planned:

- Call your diabetes care provider **AFTER** you find out the time of the surgery and if eating food in usual amounts will be allowed.

- Take your own diabetes supplies with you to the surgery:

  - blood sugar meter and strips, with finger poker (lancet)

  - insulin and syringes

  - glucose (dextrose) tablets or gel

  - blood ketone strips and meter or urine Ketostix

  - glucagon emergency kit

  - if on a pump, equipment to change insertion if needed

- Take your phone card with your diabetes care provider's numbers.

- If you/your child received a basal insulin (e.g., by insulin pump or by Lantus or Levemir injection), the basal insulin can be continued during the period of surgery. Then restart bolus pump therapy or other insulin injections when the person is able to eat.

## Table 1
# MANAGEMENT OF VOMITING (WITHOUT KETONES)

Avoid solid foods until the vomiting has stopped.

If vomiting is frequent, some doctors recommend giving a Phenergan suppository, or orally dissolved tablets called Zofran, to reduce vomiting, and wait to give fluids for an hour until the suppository is working (children under two years of age should not use a Phenergan suppository).

If you do not have suppositories, ask for a prescription for them at the time of your clinic visit.

Gradually start liquids (juice, Pedialyte®, water, etc.) in small amounts. Juices (especially orange) replace the salts that are lost with vomiting or diarrhea. Pedialyte popsicles are also available.

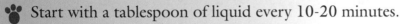 Start with a tablespoon of liquid every 10-20 minutes.

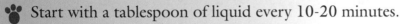 If the blood sugar is below 100 mg/dl (5.5 mmol/L):

- Sugar pop can be given.

- For some children, sucking on a piece of hard candy often works well.

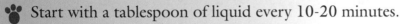 If the blood sugar is below 70 mg/dl (3.9 mmol/L) and the person is vomiting, give glucagon just as you would give insulin. The dose is 1 unit per year of age up to 15 units. Repeat doses can be given every 20 minutes as needed.

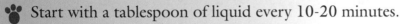 If the blood sugar is above 150 mg/dl (8.3 mmol/L), do not give pop with sugar in it.

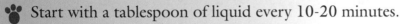 If there is no further vomiting, gradually increase the amount of fluid.

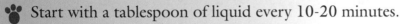 If vomiting restarts, it may again be necessary to rest the stomach for another hour and then restart the small amounts of fluids. A repeat suppository or Zofran tablet can be given after three or four hours.

After a few hours without vomiting, gradually return to a normal diet. Soups are often good to start with and they provide needed nutrients.

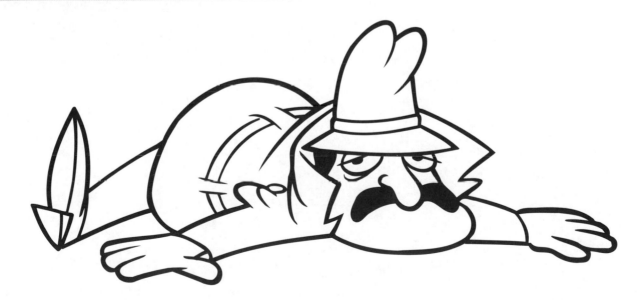

## Table 2
# SICK-DAY FOODS

**1** **Liquids***

- Fruit juice: apple, cranberry, grape, grapefruit, orange, pineapple, etc.
- Sugar-containing beverages: regular 7Up®, ginger ale, orange juice, cola, PEPSI®, etc.*
- Fruit-flavored drinks: regular Kool-Aid, lemonade, Hi-C®, etc.*
- Sports drinks: Gatorade, POWERADE®, etc., any flavor
- Tea with honey or sugar
- Pedialyte, or Infalyte® (especially for younger children)
- JELL-O®: regular (for infants, liquid JELL-O warmed in a bottle) or diet
- Popsicles, regular or diet
- Broth-type soup: bouillon, chicken noodle soup, Cup-a-Soup®

**2** **Solids** (when ready)

- Saltine crackers
- Banana (or other fruit)
- Applesauce
- Bread or toast
- Graham crackers
- Soup

*Sugar free may be needed depending on blood sugars (e.g., greater than 150 mg/dl [8.3 mmol/L]).

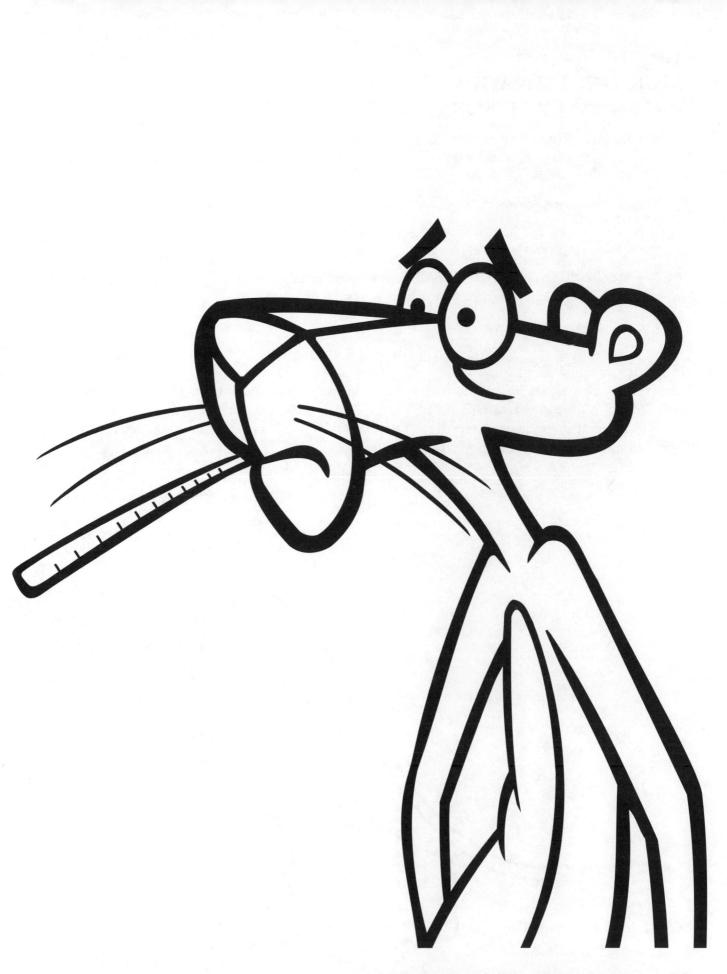

**Table 3**

# SICK-DAY MANAGEMENT: WHEN TO CALL FOR EMERGENCY CARE

- If you have vomited more than three times and can keep nothing in your stomach, and urine ketones are not moderate or large or blood ketones above 1.0 mmol/L, call your primary care physician.

- *If help is needed with an insulin dose, call your diabetes care provider.*

- If moderate or large ketones are present or blood ketones are above 1.0 mmol/L, call your diabetes care provider.

- If you have difficulty breathing or have "deep breathing," you need to go to an emergency room. This usually indicates severe acidosis (ketoacidosis).

- Low blood sugar (hypoglycemia):

If there is any unusual behavior such as confusion, slurred speech, double vision, inability to move or talk, or jerking, someone should give sugar or instant glucose. (Glucagon [Chapter 6] is given if the person is unconscious or if a convulsion [seizure] occurs.) The diabetes care provider should be contacted if a severe reaction occurs. In case of a convulsion or loss of consciousness, it may be necessary to call the paramedics or to go to an emergency room. Have an emergency number posted by the phone.

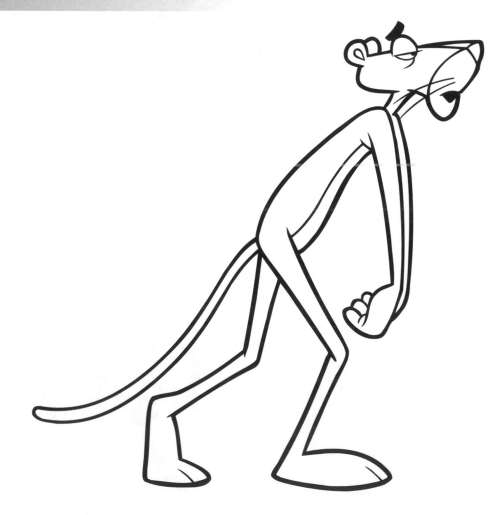

Your insulin dose may
change when you are sick,
but you always need some insulin.

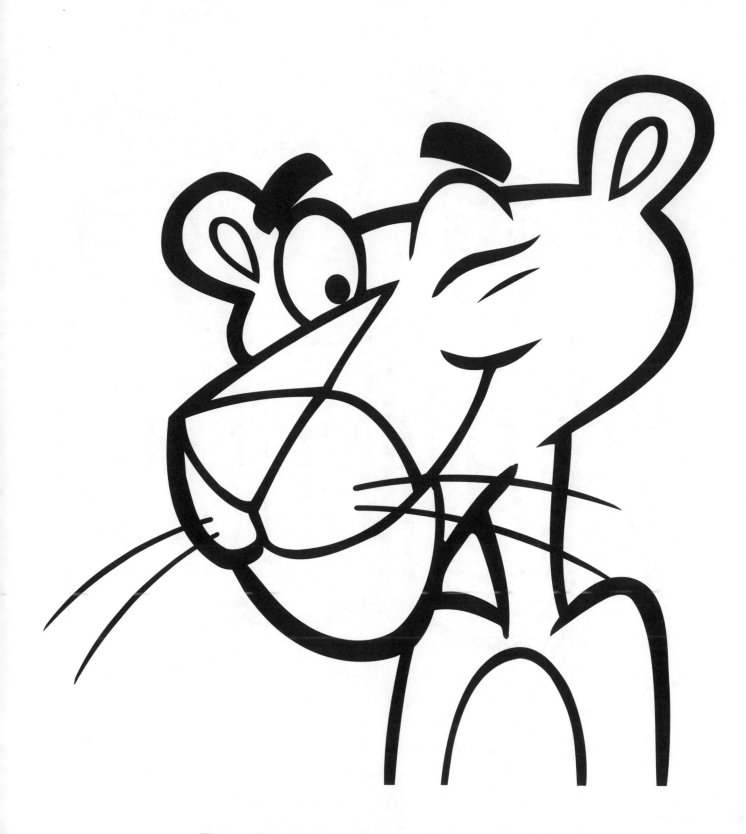

Family support is very important
for the child with diabetes.

# Chapter 17
# Family Concerns

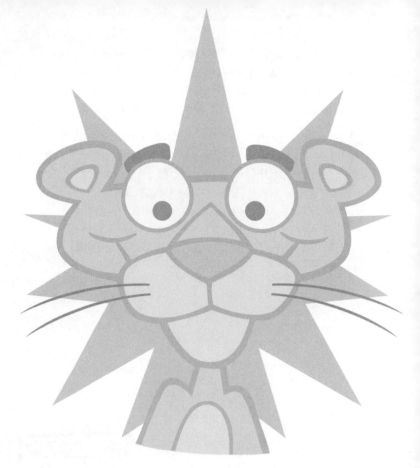

Diabetes is a family disease. This means that all family members must help. The children who do best with their diabetes have the help and support of their parents and family members.

 It is important for children with diabetes to be treated just like other children. A good rule to follow is:

THINK OF THE CHILD FIRST AND THEN THE DIABETES.

 It is important that all family members share their feelings (see Chapter 10).

 Siblings often feel left out when the child with diabetes needs more attention.

 This should be discussed with the other children and time should be set aside for them as well.

 Perhaps the most supportive and loving act that parents, brothers and sisters can make for the person with diabetes is to remove high-sugar foods (candy, sugar pop, donuts, cookies, etc.) from the home. These foods have little nutritional value. If they are around, they may be eaten without taking extra insulin, which will raise the blood sugar.

## SPECIFIC AREAS OF CONCERN

 The stress of the diagnosis of diabetes is real for all family members.

One of the four big influences on blood sugar levels is stress (see Chapter 14). The social worker or psychologist is available to help in dealing with stress.

 Extra excitement and activity may cause a low blood sugar in children with diabetes. Some of these activities can include:

- family picnics
- sleepovers
- trips to the beach or hiking
- school field days or trips
- a trip to Disney® or other theme parks
- special days such as Christmas or Hanukkah

Thinking ahead and reducing the insulin dose and giving extra snacks may result in a better day for everyone. Wearing an ID bracelet is particularly important on trips.

 Needle fears occur in about one-fourth of all people. The psychosocial team may be helpful, particularly in suggesting distractions (TV, toys, books) or relaxation techniques. The Inject-Ease device (B-D) or the use of the Insuflon (Chapter 9) is also sometimes helpful.

 Missed shots (or insulin boluses for the pumper) result in an elevated HbA$^{1c}$ level and an increased risk for diabetic complications. Help from other family members, teachers or friends may be needed.

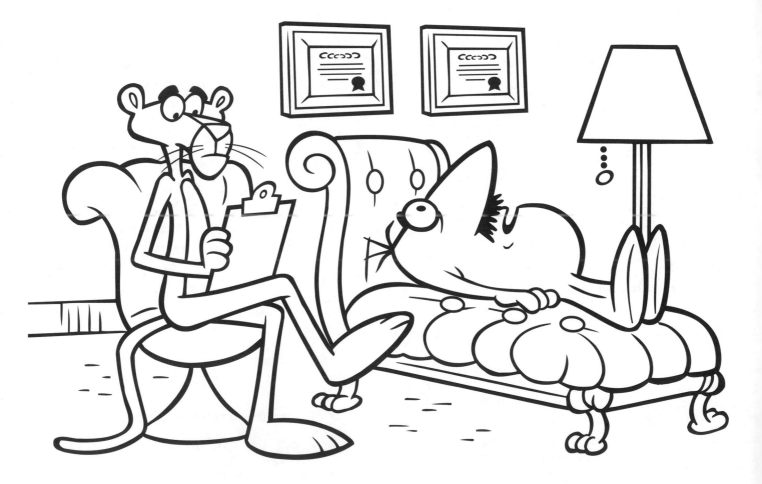

Social workers and psychologists are there to help you.

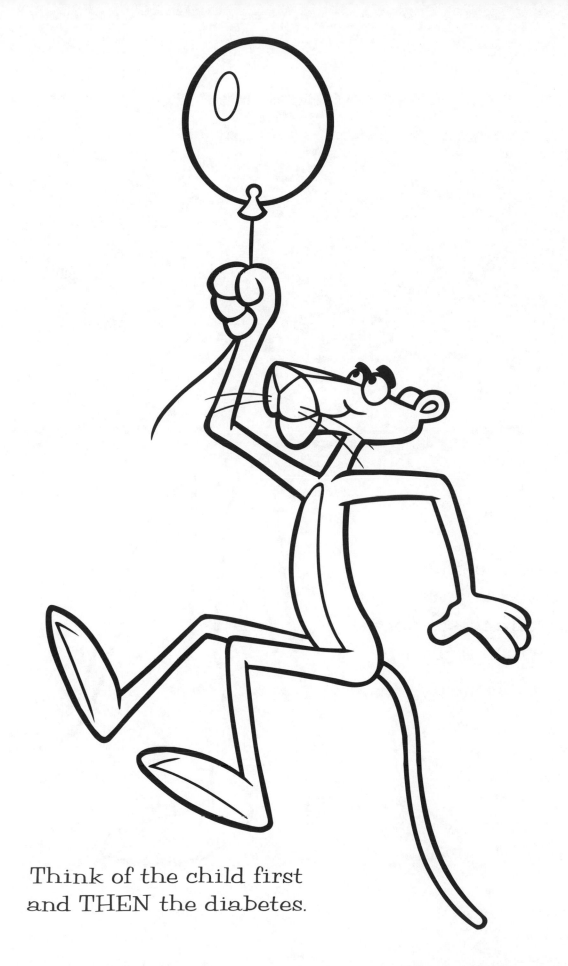

Think of the child first
and THEN the diabetes.

2 + 2 =

High or low
blood sugars
may affect school
performance.

# Chapter 18
# Responsibilities of Children at Different Ages

Children of different ages are able to handle different tasks and responsibilities. These may vary from day to day and week to week. This is true for diabetes-related tasks and non-diabetes tasks. It can be helpful for family members to have an idea of what to expect at different ages.

(See the tables of age-responsibilities in *Understanding Diabetes*, Chapter 18.)

**Below age 8 years**

 Parents do all tasks.

 Children gradually learn to cooperate.

 Shots are often given after meals or snacks (rather than before) depending upon what was eaten.

**Ages 8-12 years**

 Children begin to give some of their own shots. A common mistake is to push for too much responsibility before the child is ready.

 Having a friend spend the night or staying at a friend's house often begins during this period. As the children are often very active and use more energy from staying up later than usual, it is best to reduce the insulin dose.

 At this age, fine motor control and the sense of accuracy needed to draw up the insulin develops.

 It is important to continue to check doses of insulin drawn by the child and the blood sugar testing meters to review their readings.

 The idea of maintaining good sugar control to prevent later diabetes complications can initially be understood around age 12 or 13 years.

**Ages 13-18 years**

One of the most difficult chores for many teens is writing the blood sugar values in a log book. It is important to do this or trends in blood sugar values will be missed. Often the parents agree to do this (with the teen's OK). It is also a way for the parents to stay involved with the diabetes care and to step back in if blood sugars are not being done.

# WHAT IS THE AGE WHEN SELF-CARE SHOULD HAPPEN?

- Children should be encouraged to assume self-care as they are able.

- There isn't a "magic" age when children should take over everything.

- If too much is expected too soon, feelings of failure and low self-esteem with poor diabetes self-care may result.

**It is now believed that a supportive adult can be valuable for any person with diabetes, no matter their age.**

An alarm watch may help to remind a child of the need for a snack, or to give a shot of insulin.

Children between
the ages of 8-14
can help to manage
their diabetes.

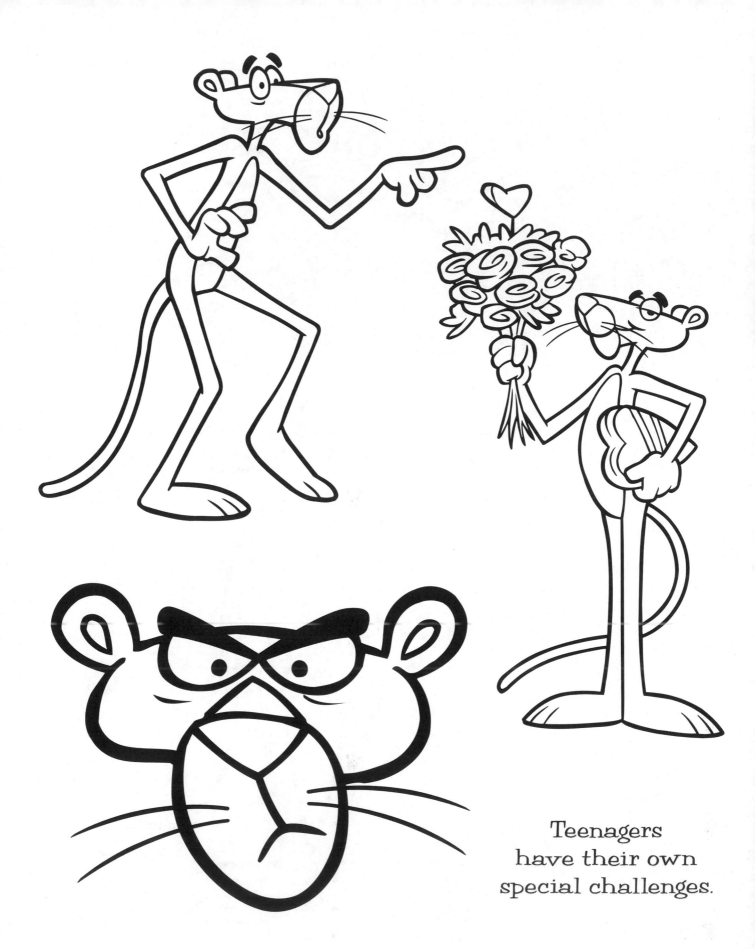

Teenagers
have their own
special challenges.

# Chapter 19
# Special Challenges of the Teen Years

The teen years are a time when young people go between wanting to be an independent adult and wanting to stay a dependent child. It is not surprising that they go back and forth when it comes to taking over the diabetes responsibilities. Many research studies now show that when parents stay involved in diabetes management, the diabetes will be in better control.

## THE CHALLENGES

- The teen-aged years are often the most difficult for having good sugar control (a good HbA$_{1c}$ level). And yet, they are important years in relation to diabetes complications.

- The teens in the intensive-treatment arm of the DCCT (Chapter 14) often had weekly clinic visits, but still had a mean HbA$_{1c}$ of 8.1% (compared with 7.1% for the adults).

- Growth and sexual hormones are at high levels and interfere with insulin activity.

- Insulin pumps, more frequent insulin shots, and the new basal insulins, insulin glargine (Lantus) or insulin detemir (Levemir) can help some teens. However, if meal shots (or boluses for pumpers) are missed, the HbA$_{1c}$ will be high.

- Driving a car safely is very important beginning in the teen years. It is important to check a blood sugar before driving. Driving with a low blood sugar can result in problems that can be just as severe as if driving while drunk.

- Diabetes is often not a priority to the teenager. Teenagers have special issues including:

  - **struggle for independence**
  - **growth and body changes**
  - **self-identity**
  - **peer relationships**
  - **sexuality**

- **consistency:** is considered a key word in diabetes management. This refers to eating, exercise, stress, or times of insulin shots. It is often hard for teens to be consistent.

- **driving a car**

- **college**

- **emotional changes**

These are all discussed in detail in the 11th edition of _Understanding Diabetes_.

🐾 **Parents must:**

- **find ways to stay involved in diabetes management.** They can be helpful in keeping the log book and in talking about insulin dosage.

- **be available to help, but should try not to be overbearing or constantly nagging.** A supportive adult can be helpful for a person with diabetes no matter their age.

🐾 **It is not surprising that diabetes is often referred to as a "disease of compromise."**

Teenagers with diabetes can lead normal lives.

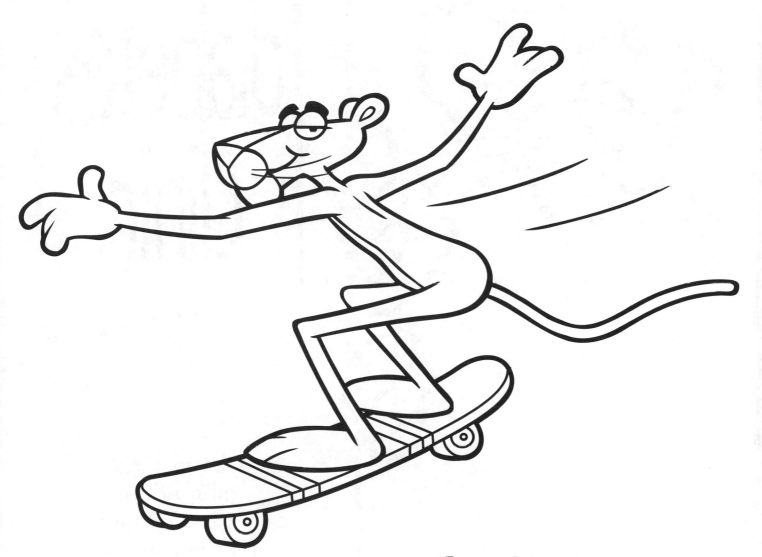

Normal teen
activities can provide
much-needed exercise.

# diabetes clinic

Clinic visits
should be
every three months
for people with
diabetes.

# Chapter 20
# Outpatient Management, Education, Support Groups, and Standards of Care

## WHAT SHOULD HAPPEN AFTER A DIAGNOSIS OF DIABETES?

- Regular follow-up visits should be every three months for people with diabetes. Diabetes education should continue for the patient and family at these visits.

- The insulin dose may be changed during these visits. It is usually increased one-half unit per pound of weight gained (just to have the same dose for weight).

- Growth and other signs of sugar control such as liver size and finger curvatures are checked. If blood sugars are high, the sugar collects on the joint proteins and finger curvatures may result.

- On the physical exam, items such as thyroid size and eye changes are checked.

- The HbA$_{1c}$ blood test (see Chapter 14) should be done every three months.

- After having diabetes for three years as a teen or adult, eye exams by an eye doctor and special kidney tests are very important to have each year (see Chapter 22).

- For people with type 2 diabetes, the eye and kidney tests should be done at the time of diagnosis, and then yearly.

## WHAT ELSE IS IMPORTANT?

- Communication (fax, e-mail) of blood sugar values to the health care provider is often helpful.

- The families should let their diabetes provider or diabetes team know about any of the following:

  - any severe low blood sugar (hypoglycemic) reactions

  - frequent mild reactions

  - moderate or large urine ketones or blood ketones above 1.0 mmol/L

79

- any planned surgery
- if at least half of the blood sugar values are not in the desired range for age (see Chapter 7)

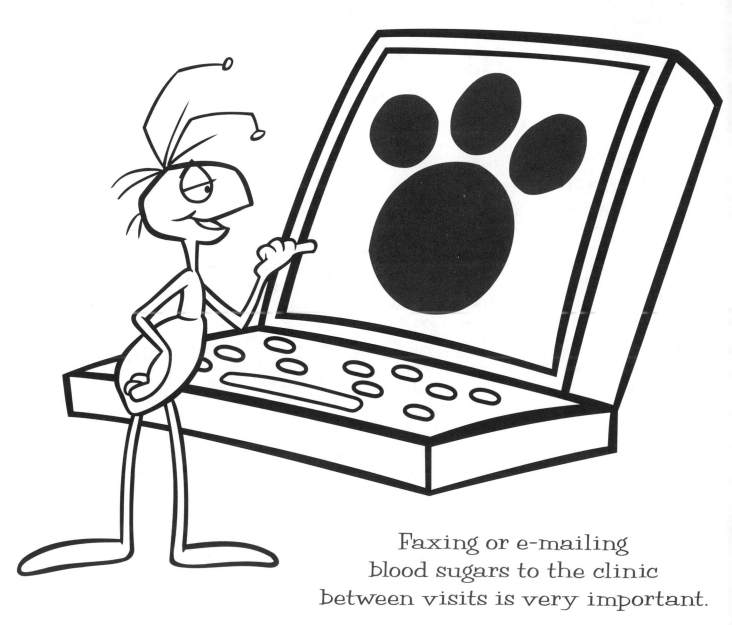

Support groups and special educational programs (Research Updates, Grandparents Workshop, College-Bound Workshop, etc.) are available in many areas.

Special events (ski trips, bike trips, camping, a Halloween party, etc.) help children and families to learn more about diabetes. They also provide a chance to talk to others who have a family member with diabetes.

Faxing or e-mailing blood sugars to the clinic between visits is very important.

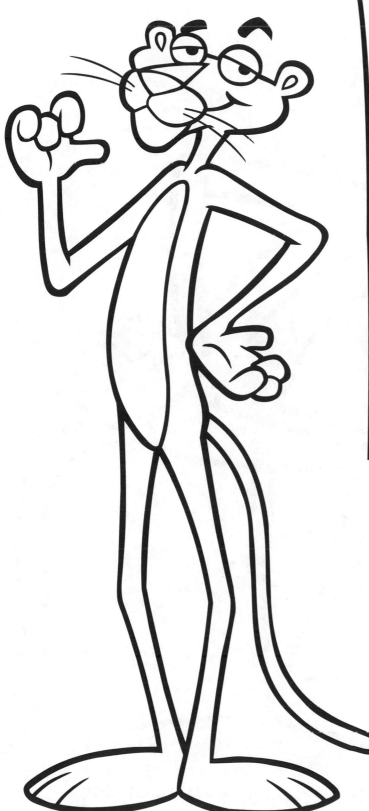

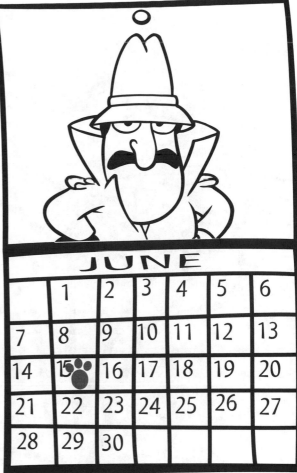

JUNE

| 1 | 2 | 3 | 4 | 5 | 6 |
|---|---|---|---|---|---|
| 7 | 8 | 9 | 10 | 11 | 12 | 13 |
| 14 | 15 | 16 | 17 | 18 | 19 | 20 |
| 21 | 22 | 23 | 24 | 25 | 26 | 27 |
| 28 | 29 | 30 | | | | |

Mark your calendar
to remind you
of follow-up visits
every three months.

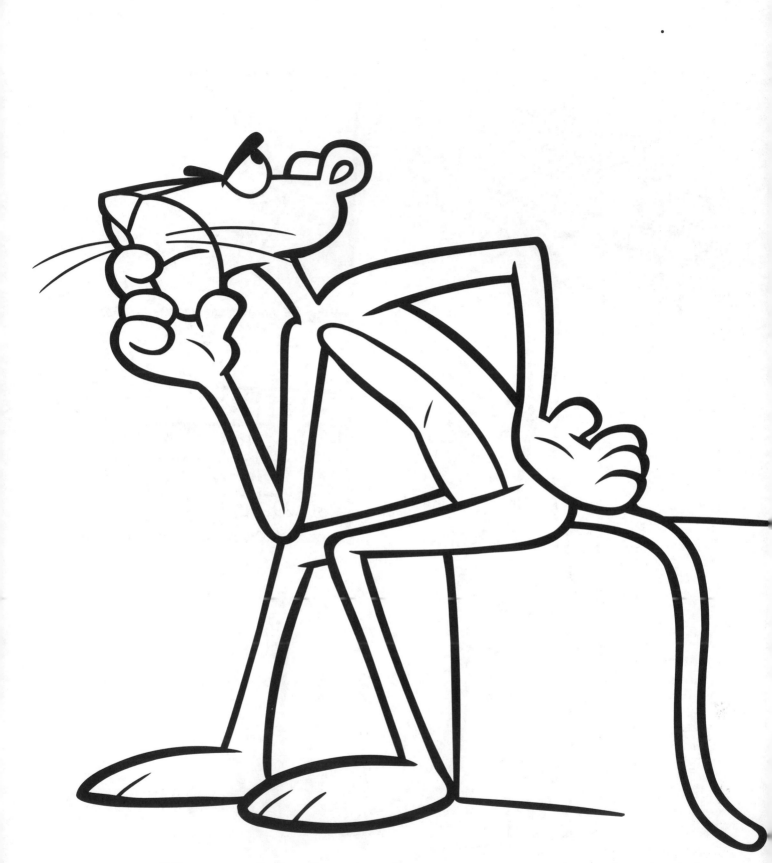

You need to think about your insulin dose.

# Chapter 21
# Adjusting the Insulin Dose, Correction Factors, and "Thinking" Scales

Six to twelve months after the diagnosis of diabetes, many families feel OK with changing the insulin doses on their own.

## HOW AND WHEN SHOULD AN INSULIN DOSE BE CHANGED?

**Below are four methods:**

1. **Looking at blood sugar patterns over the last week:**

🐾 It is necessary to know which insulin is acting at the time of the highs or lows in order to make the correct changes (see figures in Chapter 8).

🐾 If more than half of the blood sugar values at any time of the day are above the desired range for the age of the person (see table in Chapter 7):

- The insulin dose acting at the time of the high sugar value should be increased.

- If values are still high after three days, the dose can be increased again.

🐾 If there are more than two lows (below 60 mg/dl [3.3 mmol/L]) at one time of day:

- The insulin dose acting at that time should be decreased.

- If more lows occur, the dose can be decreased again the next day.

🐾 With small children, the change in dose may be by one half to one unit.

🐾 With older children and teens, the change in dose may be by one or two units.

🐾 Blood sugars will be lowest the first day after an increase in insulin and highest the first day after a decrease in insulin.

🐾 Tables are given in the larger book, _Understanding Diabetes_ (Chapter 21) for people wanting more detailed suggestions on changing insulin doses for high or low blood sugars.

## 2. Using a "correction factor":

🐾 Some people use a combination of a **"correction factor"** and carbohydrate (carb) counting (see Chapter 12) to determine the dose of rapid-acting insulin before meals and snacks.

🐾 The **correction factor** can be used to "correct" a high blood sugar down to a target blood sugar level (e.g., 150 mg/dl [8.3 mmol/L]).

🐾 The most common **correction factor** is to give one unit of insulin for every 50 mg/dl (2.8 mmol/L) of glucose above 150 mg/dl (8.3 mmol/L), e.g., if the blood sugar is 250 mg/dl (13.9 mmol/L), the correction factor would be 2 units. Many teens correct down to 120 mg/dl (6.7 mmol/L) or even 100 mg/dl (5.5 mmol/L) during the day. However, every person is different and the **correction factor** should be adjusted to fit the individual.

🐾 At bedtime, during the night, or before exercise, the correction factor is usually reduced by half.

🐾 It is generally wise to wait two hours between correction insulin dosages.

## 3. Using "thinking" scales:

🐾 The insulin dose is figured by considering many factors, including:

- the blood sugar level
- illness
- any exercise that has been or is to be done
- stress
- food to be eaten
- menses

## 4. Changes for Lantus or Levemir:

🐾 Adjustments are usually made based on the morning (fasting) sugar level.

🐾 Doses are increased or decreased if blood sugar levels are above or below the recommended values for age (see Chapter 7).

🐾 As suggested above, dose changes for a young child may be by one half to one unit, and for older children (and teens), by one to two units.

🐾 Suggested waiting times between dose changes are as given above.

## Table
# Example of Insulin Adjustments

| Blood Sugar | | Correction Factor* | Carb Choices** | Total Units |
| mg/dl | mmol/L | Units of Insulin | (15g carb) | of Insulin |
| --- | --- | --- | --- | --- |
| Less than 150 | 8.3 | 0 | 1 | 1 |
| 200 | 11.1 | 1 | 2 | 3 |
| 250 | 13.9 | 2 | 3 | 5 |
| 300 | 16.7 | 3 | 4 | 7 |
| 350 | 19.4 | 4 | 5 | 9 |

*Assuming a correction factor of 1 unit of rapid-acting insulin per 50 mg/dl (2.8 mmol/L) above 150 mg/dl (8.3 mmol/L).

** One carb choice = 15g carbohydrate. In this example, 1 unit of insulin is given for each 15g carb choice. In the U.K., carb choices are usually 10g of carbohydrates.

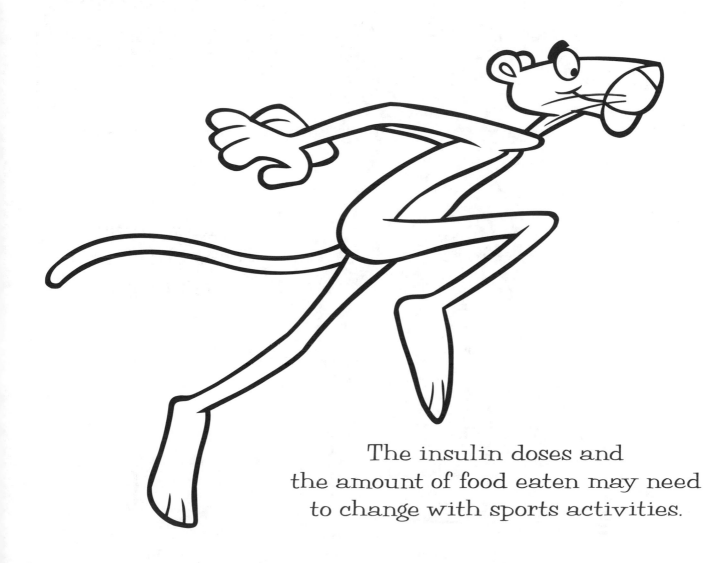

The insulin doses and the amount of food eaten may need to change with sports activities.

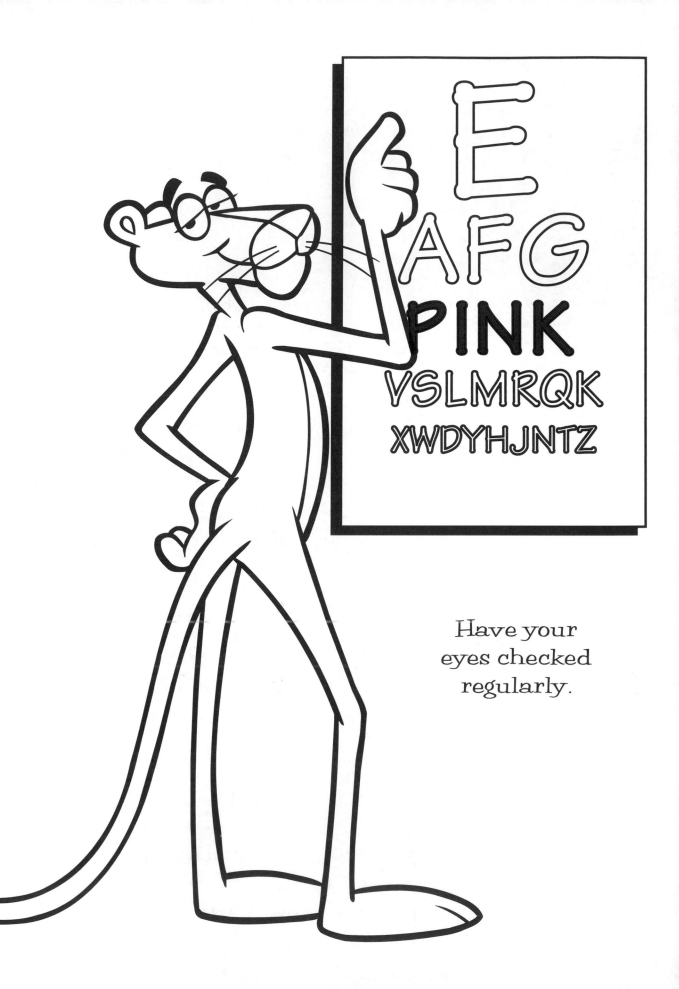

E
AFG
PINK
VSLMRQK
XWDYHJNTZ

Have your
eyes checked
regularly.

# Chapter 22
# Long-Term Complications of Diabetes

## WHAT CAN MAKE THE RISK OF THESE COMPLICATIONS LESS?

🐾 Good sugar control will reduce the risk for eye, kidney, nerve, and heart complications of diabetes by more than 50 percent as shown by the DCCT (Chapter 14).

🐾 Not smoking (or chewing) tobacco also helps.

🐾 Another factor is the blood pressure. Researchers at our Center showed that even mild increases in blood pressure are bad for the eyes and kidneys.

## HOW ARE COMPLICATIONS FOUND?

**Small blood vessel problems:**

• Eye exams (and sometimes photographs) by the eye doctor tell if someone is developing eye damage.

• The *microalbumin* test tells if someone is getting early kidney damage at a time when it may still be reversible. The instructions for doing the microalbumin test to detect early kidney damage are at the end of Chapter 22 in *Understanding Diabetes*. We prefer overnight urine collections because a false positive result is less likely.

• Screening tests for the eyes and kidneys should be done once yearly for people who have had type 1 diabetes for three or more years and have reached puberty (age 10 to 12 years).

• People who have type 2 diabetes should have the eye and kidney tests done soon after diagnosis and then every year.

• Families may need to help remind the health care team that it is time to do the microalbumin test or to see an eye doctor.

• Treatment of early eye or kidney damage is done by improving sugar control.

• Treatment of early kidney damage is also done by lowering blood pressure. A blood pressure medicine called an ACE-inhibitor is often helpful.

• If many eye changes are present, laser treatment to the back of the eye (retina) may help to prevent more severe problems.

**Large blood vessel problems in adults:**

- Heart attacks and other blood vessel diseases are a greater risk for adults with diabetes.

- Cholesterol levels and a lipid panel should be checked yearly.

- A baby aspirin and/or a fish oil capsule (omega-3 fatty acid) taken once or twice daily may help in prevention.

## TWO OTHER DISEASES THAT CAN OCCUR IN PEOPLE WITH DIABETES ARE:

1. **Thyroid problems:** thyroid problems (like type 1 diabetes) are due to autoimmunity (see Chapter 3). Antibodies are made against the thyroid gland.

2. **Celiac disease:** this is an allergy to the wheat protein, gluten. It occurs in 1 of every 20 people with diabetes. There may be stomach complaints (pain, gas, diarrhea) or poor growth. Half of the people with celiac disease have no symptoms. The treatment is to remove all wheat, rye and barley products from the diet. Meeting with a dietitian is important. Websites for obtaining more information on celiac disease and foods to avoid are given in *"Understanding Diabetes."*

Finger curvatures can be a sign of high blood sugar levels over many years.

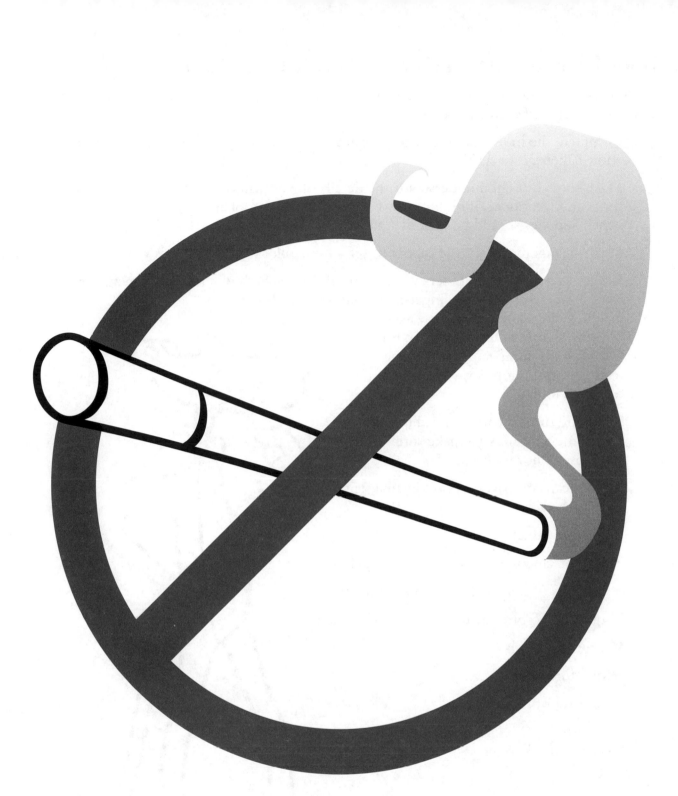

# DO NOT SMOKE!
## (or chew tobacco!)

# School Diabetes Management Checklist for Parents

_____ Discuss specific care of your child with the teachers, school nurse, bus driver, coaches and other staff who will be involved.

_____ Complete the individualized school health care plan with the help of school staff and your diabetes care staff.

_____ Make sure your child understands the details of who will help him/her with testing, shots and treatment of high or low blood sugars at school and where supplies will be kept. Supplies should be kept in a place where they are always available if needed.

_____ Make arrangements for the school to send home blood sugar records weekly.

_____ Keep current phone numbers where you can be reached. Collect equipment for school: meter, strips and finger-poker, lancets, insulin, insulin syringes or pen, biohazard container, log book or a copy of testing record form, extra insulin pump supplies, ketone testing strips, photo for substitute teacher's folder.

_____ Food and drinks; parents need to check intermittently to make sure supplies are not used up:

  ▼ juice cans or boxes (approximately 15g of carb each)

  ▼ glucose tablets

  ▼ instant glucose or cake decorating gel

  ▼ crackers (± peanut butter and/or cheese)

  ▼ quarters to buy sugar pop (soda) if needed

  ▼ Fruit Roll-Ups

  ▼ dried fruit

  ▼ raisins or other snacks

_____ Box with the child's name to store these food and drink items

## Chapter 23
# The School and Diabetes

Parents want to know that their child is in safe hands while at school. It is the parents' responsibility (not the child's) to inform and educate the school. Parents also want to make sure their child is not treated differently as a result of having diabetes.

## WHAT SHOULD BE DONE?

🐾 Many schools now require school health plans. An individualized school health plan (which you are welcome to copy) is included in this chapter. The parents and diabetes nurse should fill this out. The parents can then go over the plan with the school nurse or aide.

🐾 The parents must also provide supplies for the school. Some children keep a separate meter and strips at the school. Others bring their home meter and supplies in their backpack. See parents checklist.

🐾 Other forms that you may want to copy from _Understanding Diabetes_ (Chapter 23) are:

1) School Intake Interview

2) Emergency Response Plan

3) Individualize Health Care Plan Check List for the School Nurse

4) Insulin Pumps in the School Setting

5) A general letter for the principal and school nurse

## WHAT CAN HAPPEN AT SCHOOL?

• Low blood sugars are the most likely emergency to occur at school. It may be helpful for the family to copy and review the table on mild, moderate and severe reactions with the school (see Chapter 6). _Supplies for treating lows will also need to be provided by the family._

• High blood sugars and/or ketones may also occur at school, particularly with stress, illness, overeating or lack of exercise. If the blood sugar is above 300 mg/dl (16.7 mmol/L) the urine or blood ketones need to be checked. When the blood sugar is high it is generally necessary to go to the bathroom more frequently. _If small to moderate urine ketones or blood ketones above 0.6 mmol/L occur, the parents need to be called._

• In addition to the forms in this chapter, _Understanding Diabetes_ has insulin pump and other school forms.

# HEALTHCARE PROVIDER ORDER FOR STUDENT WITH DIABETES

Student _____ DOB _____ School _____ Grade _____

Doctor _____ Phone _____ Diabetes Educator _____ Phone _____

**Monitor Blood Glucose**  ☐ Before lunch  ☐ After lunch  ☐ Before PE  ☐ After PE  ☐ Before snack

☐ Before getting on bus/driving home   ☐ As needed for signs/symptoms of low or high blood glucose

Notify parent when blood sugar <_____ or >_____.   Target range for blood sugar >_____mg/dl to <_____.

## Hypoglycemia  Student should not be sent to office unaccompanied if symptomatic or BS < _____ mg/dl.

✓ Check blood glucose - if blood glucose meters not available, treat symptoms.

✓ Blood glucose between _____ mg/dl and symptomatic: Treat with juice or glucose tabs.

✓ Mild symptoms: Treat with juice, glucose tabs, etc. until above _____ mg/dl, then 10 to 15 gram carbohydrate snack or lunch.

✓ Moderate symptoms if unable to drink juice: Administer glucose gel. Retreat until above _____mg/dl, then snack or l.

✓ Severe symptoms which may include seizures, unconscious, unable or unwilling to take gel or juice:
Administer Glucagon ___ mg(s) ☐ IM or _____ units on insulin syringe  ☐ SQ if trained staff available and call 911.

## Hyperglycemia

☐ Check urine ketones if blood glucose is over 300 mg/dl or with symptoms of illness/vomiting. If ketones present, call parents, provide water and student should not exercise. Student may need insulin via injection.

☐ Use sliding scale insulin orders when blood glucose is _____mg/dl.

✓ Recommend student be released from school when ketones are moderate/large or symptoms of illness in order to be treated and monitored more closely by parent/guardian.

## Medication

Student is on ☐ oral diabetes medication(s)  Dose: _____  **Times to be given** _____

Student is on ☐ insulin. Type:_____  Dose: _____  **Times to be given** _____

**Blood Glucose Correction and Insulin Dosage using (Rapid Acting) Insulin:**  _____

Blood Glucose Range _____ mg/dl  Administer _____ units

Blood Glucose Range _____ mg/dl  Administer _____ units

Blood Glucose Range _____ mg/dl  Administer _____ units

Blood Glucose Range _____ mg/dl  Administer _____ units and check ketones

Blood Glucose Range _____ mg/dl  Administer _____ units and check ketones

Blood Glucose Range _____ mg/dl  Administer _____ units and check ketones

Blood Glucose  Range_____ mg/dl  Administer _____ units and check ketones

If ketones present, call parents, provide water and student should not exercise.

Carbohydrate counting _____ unit(s) of insulin per _____ grams of carbohydrate with lunch.

☐ Parent/guardian authorized to increase or decrease sliding scale within the following range: +/- 2 units of insulin.

☐ Parent/guardian authorized to increase or decrease insulin to carbohydrate ratio within the following range: 1 unit per prescribed grams of carbohydrates +/- 5 grams of carbohydrates.

## Student's Self Care  (ability level) to be completed by parent

| | | | | |
|---|---|---|---|---|
| Totally independent management. | ☐ Yes ☐ No | Self injects with trained staff supervision. | ☐ Yes ☐ No |
| Monitors independently. | ☐ Yes ☐ No | Injections to be done by trained staff. | ☐ Yes ☐ No |
| Needs verification of blood glucose by staff. | ☐ Yes ☐ No | Self treats mild hypoglycemia. | ☐ Yes ☐ No |
| Assist/testing to be done by trained staff. | ☐ Yes ☐ No | Monitors own snacks and meals. | ☐ Yes ☐ No |
| Administers insulin independently. | ☐ Yes ☐ No | Independently counts carbohydrates. | ☐ Yes ☐ No |
| Self injects with verification of dose. | ☐ Yes ☐ No | Monitors and interprets urine/blood ketones. | ☐ Yes ☐ No |

## SIGNATURES

My signature below provides authorization for the above written orders and exchange of health information to assist the school nurse in developing an Individualized Health Plan. I understand that all procedures will be implemented in accordance with state laws and regulations and may be performed by unlicensed designated school personnel under the training and supervision provided by the school nurse. This order is for a maximum of one year.

Physician _____   Date _____

Parent _____   Date _____

School Nurse _____   Date _____

# HEALTHCARE PROVIDER ORDER FOR STUDENT WITH DIABETES ON PUMP

Student _____ DOB _____ School _____ Grade _____

Doctor _____ Phone _____ Diabetes Educator _____ Phone_____

**Pump settings are established by the student's healthcare provider and should not be changed by school staff.**

**Monitor Blood Glucose** ☐ Before lunch   ☐ After lunch   ☐ Before PE   ☐ After PE   ☐ Before snack
☐ Before getting on bus/driving home   ☐ As needed for signs/symptoms of low or high blood glucose

Notify parent when blood sugar <_____ or >_____.     Target range for blood sugar >_____ mg/dl to <_____.

---

## Hypoglycemia   Student should not be sent to office unaccompanied if symptomatic or BS < _____ mg/dl.

✓ Check blood glucose - if blood glucose meters not available, treat symptoms.

✓ Blood glucose between _____ mg/dl and symptomatic: Treat with 10 to 15 gram carbohydrate snack.

✓ Mild symptoms: Treat with juice, glucose tabs, etc. until above _____ mg/dl, then snack or lunch.

✓ Moderate symptoms if unable to drink juice: Administer glucose gel. Retreat until above _____ mg/dl, then snack or l.

✓ Severe symptoms which may include seizures, unconscious, unable or unwilling to take gel or juice:
Administer Glucagon _____ mg(s) ☐ IM or _____ units on insulin syringe ☐ SQ if trained staff available and call 911.
Disconnect pump.

**Do not bolus for carbohydrates given to treat low blood glucose** until blood glucose is > 70 mg/dl.

## Hyperglycemia

☐ If BS >300 mg/dl with ketones or 2 consecutive unexplained BS >300 mg/dl (with or without ketones), i.e. malfunctioning pump. Student may require insulin via injection and/or new infusion site/set.

☐ First contact parent then healthcare provider for further instructions may need insulin via syringe.

Check ☐ Urine ☐ Blood ketones if blood glucose > _____ mg/dl

• If ketones present, call parents, provide water and student should not exercise.

• Recommend student be released from school when ketones are moderate/large or symptoms of illness in order to be treated and monitored more closely by parent/guardian.

## Insulin dosing for High Blood Glucose and/or Carbs

☐ Blood glucose correction when blood sugar >_____ and insulin dosage via syringe is only to be administered when confirmed by school nurse, parent or healthcare provider for treatment of hyperglycemia: Insulin – Type: _____

Blood Glucose Range _____ mg/dl   Administer _____ units
Blood Glucose Range _____ mg/dl   Administer _____ units
Blood Glucose Range _____ mg/dl   Administer _____ units
Blood Glucose Range _____ mg/dl   Administer _____ units and check ketones
Blood Glucose Range _____ mg/dl   Administer _____ units and check ketones
Blood Glucose Range _____ mg/dl   Administer _____ units and check ketones
Blood Glucose  Range _____ mg/dl   Administer _____ units and check ketones

---

Insulin to Carbohydrate ratio _____ units of insulin per _____ grams of carbohydrate.

Carbohydrate ratio for snack _____ units per _____ gm of carbs   _____ am   _____ pm

Bolus for carbohydrates (or to be) eaten should occur immediately ☐ Before lunch ☐ After lunch ☐ ½ bolus before & ½ bolus after

---

**Student's Self Care:** (ability level)

| | | | | |
|---|---|---|---|---|
| Independently monitors blood glucose. | ☐ Yes ☐ No | Troubleshoots all alarms. | ☐ Yes ☐ No | |
| Independently counts carbohydrates. | ☐ Yes ☐ No | Administers insulin independently. | ☐ Yes ☐ No | |
| Needs assistance with pump management. | ☐ Yes ☐ No | Self injects with verification of dosage. | ☐ Yes ☐ No | |
| Independently manages pump boluses. | ☐ Yes ☐ No | Injection to be done by trained staff | ☐ Yes ☐ No | |
| Inserts new infusion set. | ☐ Yes ☐ No | Self treats mild hypoglycemia. | ☐ Yes ☐ No | |
| | | Tests and interprets urine/blood ketones. | ☐ Yes ☐ No | |

---

## SIGNATURES

My signature below provides authorization for the above written orders and exchange of health information to assist the school nurse in developing an Individualized Health Plan. I understand that all procedures will be implemented in accordance with state laws and regulations and may be performed by unlicensed designated school personnel under the training and supervision provided by the school nurse. This order is for a maximum of one year.

Physician _____   Date _____

Parent _____   Date _____

School Nurse _____   Date _____

STUDENT: _____ DOB: _____

# EMERGENCY RESPONSE PLAN

## MILD LOW BLOOD SUGAR: (Hypoglycemia) — (IF STUDENT IS ALERT)
Student to be treated when blood sugar is below:_____.
Symptoms could include: hunger, irritability, shakiness, sleepiness, sweating, pallor, uncooperative, or other behavior changes
Additional symptoms: _____

**Treatment of Mild:** With any level of low blood sugar **never** leave the student unattended. If treatment is required outside the classroom, **a responsible person should <u>accompany</u> student to the health clinic or office** for further assistance.
Test blood sugar. **<u>If kit is not available,</u>** treat child immediately for low blood sugar
If blood sugar is between _____and _____ and lunch is available, <u>escort</u> to lunch and have child eat **immediately!**
If lunch is unavailable, treat immediately as listed below.
If blood sugar is below_____ , give _____oz of juice or (1/3 can) regular sugar pop or _____ glucose tablets.
Retest in 10 minutes. If still below_____ retreat as above.
When blood sugar rises above_____ or when symptoms improve provide snack or lunch.
Notify parent/guardian and school nurse.
Comments: _____

## MODERATE LOW BLOOD SUGAR: (IF STUDENT IS NOT ALERT AND NOT ABLE TO SELF TREAT)
Symptoms: In addition to those listed above for mild low blood sugar, student may be **combative, disoriented or incoherent, slurred speech**
**Treatment for Moderate Low Blood Sugar:**
**If student is conscious yet <u>unable</u> to self-administer or drink the fluids offered:**
✓ Administer ¾ to 1 tube (3 tsp) of glucose gel, or ¾ tube to 1 tube of cake decorating gel. **<u>Will need to treat with gel until child is</u> <u>alert!</u>** ✓ Place between cheek and gums and massage, elevate head and encourage student to swallow. Student may be uncooperative.
✓ Notify parent/guardian and school nurse.
✓ Retest in 10 minutes. If still below _____ retreat as above.
Comments: _____

## SEVERE LOW BLOOD SUGAR:
Symptoms: **<u>Seizure, loss of consciousness, or unable/unwilling to take gel or juice.</u>**
✓ **Stay with student**       ✓ **Roll student on side**     ✓ **Do not put anything in mouth**
✓ **Appoint someone to call 911**     ✓ **Protect from injury**     ✓ **Contact parent/guardian and school nurse**
Give Glucagon subcutaneously (if ordered and if a nurse or other delegated person is available); dose = _____mg  or _____units
**(1.0mg=100 units, 0.5mg=50 units, 0.25mg=25 units, 10 units for < 2yrs.)**
**mg to be used  with intramuscular syringe and units to be used with insulin syringe.**
**Instructions for mixing glucagon: mix liquid from syringe into vial and draw up the appropriate dose.**
      (if child is under the age of 6 yrs, may use insulin syringe to administer dose)
Comments: _____

## HIGH BLOOD SUGAR: Student needs to be treated when blood sugar is above _____.
Call parent or guardian when blood sugar is greater than _____.
Symptoms could include (circle all that apply): extreme thirst, headache, abdominal pain, nausea, increased urination
Additional symptoms: _____
**<u>Treatment for High Blood Sugar:</u>**
Student needs to drink increased amounts of fluids and must       ✓ Be allowed to carry water bottle       ✓ Be allowed to use restroom
drink _____oz water or DIET pop  (caffeine free) <u>every hour</u>.                                                    as often as needed
**(Amount of fluid should equal to 1oz per year of age, up to 16 oz. max)**

Check urine or blood ketones, if blood sugar is greater than _____2x or when ill/and or vomiting. If urine ketones are **moderate to large or if blood ketones are greater than 0.6 mmol, call parent/guardian immediately! Do not allow exercise.**
**Administer insulin if ordered and if trained personnel available.**
**When ketones are moderate-large, recommend child be released from school in order to be treated and monitored more closely by parent/guardian.**
**If student exhibits nausea, vomiting, stomachache or lethargy, contact parent/guardian, student should be released from school.**
**Send student back to class if none of the above physical symptoms are present.**

## SIGNATURES
My signature below provides authorization for the above written orders and exchange of health information to assist the school nurse in developing an Individualized Health Plan.  I understand that all procedures will be implemented in accordance with state laws and regulations and may be performed by unlicensed designated school personnel under the training and supervision provided by the school nurse. This order is for a maximum of one year.

Physician _____     Date _____

Parent _____     Date _____

School Nurse _____     Date _____

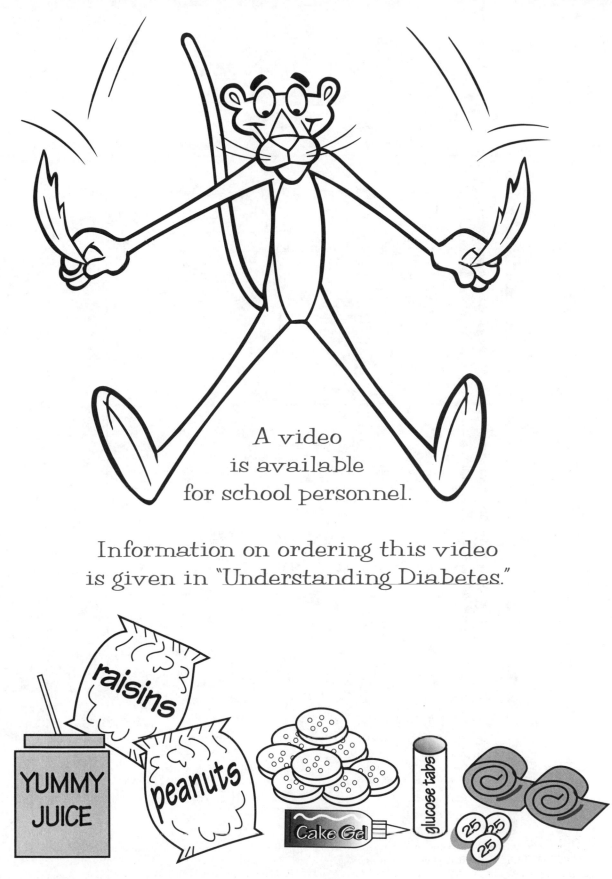

A video
is available
for school personnel.

Information on ordering this video
is given in "Understanding Diabetes."

Make sure that you have snacks handy at school
in case you need them.

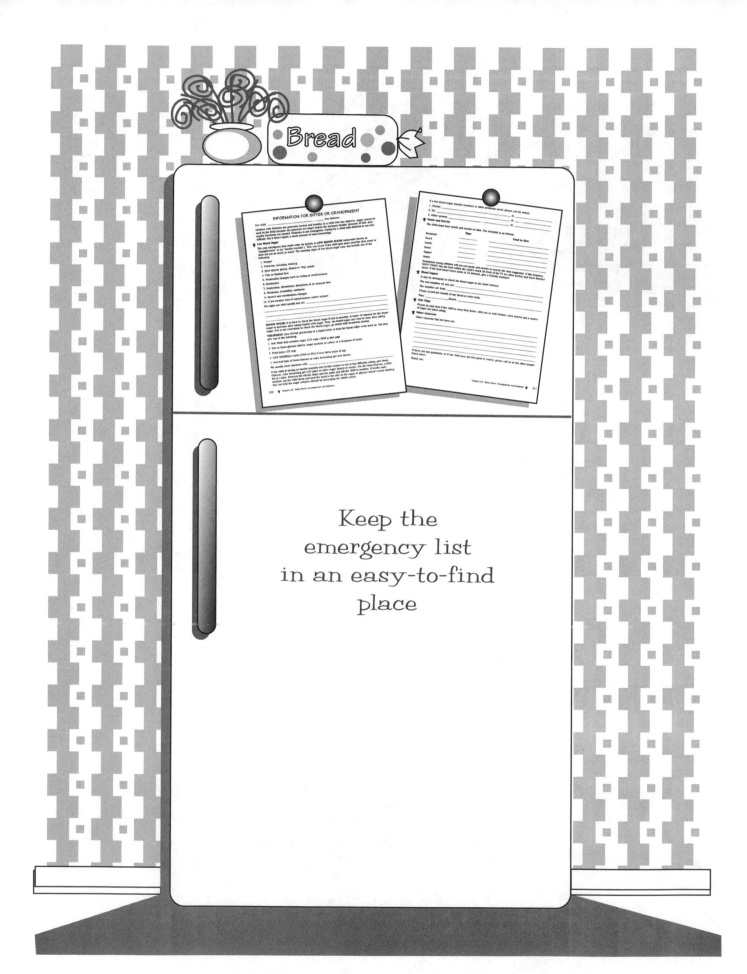

Keep the
emergency list
in an easy-to-find
place

# Chapter 24
# Baby-sitters, Grandparents, and Other Caregivers

It is important for parents to feel that their child is safe with caregivers other than the parents. It is also important for these caregivers to feel confident that they can do a good job.

## WHAT DO THEY NEED TO KNOW?

🐾 How much training is needed will depend upon the amount of time the child will be with the caregiver, and the age of the child.

All caregivers need:

• some information about signs of low blood sugar and how to treat it. A low blood sugar can occur at any time.

• some basic instruction on foods and diabetes. A two-page handout is in this chapter, which can be cut out or copied for the caregiver.

• emergency phone numbers in case the parents cannot be reached. This helps everyone feel better.

• to know how to give shots, when to check for urine or blood ketones, and other more detailed information if the parents are to be away for a longer time period.

• an extra supply of insulin, etc. (in case a bottle is dropped and broken).

🐾 Attending a "Grandparent Workshop" or other workshop can help to teach the grandparents, baby-sitters or other caregivers about diabetes.

• It is important for the child and the grandparents to continue to have a close relationship.

• It can also help to remove any fears about giving shots or treating low blood sugars.

🐾 Caregivers may wish to join the parents at initial education classes or at the time of clinic visits. They are always welcome.

# Information for the Sitter or Grandparent

Our child, _____, has diabetes.

Children with diabetes are generally normal and healthy. In a child who has diabetes, sugar cannot be used by the body because the pancreas no longer makes the hormone insulin. Because of this, daily insulin injections are needed. Diabetes is not contagious. Caring for a child with diabetes is not very difficult, but it does require a small amount of extra knowledge.

### Low Blood Sugar

The only emergency that could come on quickly is **LOW BLOOD SUGAR** (otherwise known as "hypoglycemia" or an "insulin reaction"). This can occur if the child gets more exercise than usual or does not eat as much as usual. *The warning signs of low blood sugar vary but include any of the following:* (They are discussed in greater detail in Chapter 6.)

1. Hunger
2. Paleness, sweating, shaking
3. Eyes appear glassy, dilated or "big" pupils
4. Pale or flushed face
5. Personality changes such as crying or stubbornness
6. Headaches
7. Inattention, drowsiness, sleepiness at an unusual time
8. Weakness, irritability, confusion
9. Speech and coordination changes
10. If not treated, loss of consciousness and/or seizure

The signs our child usually has are: _____

_____

_____

**BLOOD SUGAR:** It is ideal to check the blood sugar if this is possible. It takes 10 minutes for the blood sugar to increase after taking liquids with sugar. Thus, the blood sugar can even be done after taking sugar. If it is not convenient to check the blood sugar, go ahead with treatment anyway.

**TREATMENT:** Give SUGAR (preferably in a liquid form) to help the blood sugar rise.

*You may give any of the following:*

1. One-half cup of soft drink that contains sugar – **NOT a diet pop**
2. Three or four glucose tablets, sugar packets or cubes
3. One-half cup of fruit juice
4. LIFE-SAVERS candy (FIVE or SIX pieces) if over three years of age
5. One-half tube of Insta-Glucose or cake decorating gel (see below)

We usually treat reactions with: _____

If the child is having an insulin reaction and he/she refuses to eat or has difficulty eating, give Insta-Glucose, cake decorating gel (1/2 tube) or other sugar (honey or syrup). Put the Insta-Glucose, a little bit at a time, between the cheeks (lips) and the gums and tell the child to swallow. If he/she can't swallow, lay the child down and turn the head to the side so the sugar or glucose doesn't cause choking. You can help the sugar solution absorb by massaging the child's cheek.

If a low blood sugar (insulin reaction) or other problems occur, please call:

1. Parent: _____ at: _____

2. _____ at: _____

3. _____ at: _____

## 🐾 Meals and Snacks

*The child must have meals and snacks on time.  The schedule is as follows:*

| | Time | Food to Give |
|---|---|---|
| Breakfast | _____ | _____ |
| Snack | _____ | _____ |
| Lunch | _____ | _____ |
| Snack | _____ | _____ |
| Supper | _____ | _____ |
| Snack | _____ | _____ |

Sometimes young children will not eat meals and snacks at exactly the time suggested.  If this happens, DON'T PANIC!  Set the food within the child's reach (in front of the TV set often works) and leave him/her alone.  If the food hasn't been eaten in 10 minutes, give a friendly reminder.  Allow about 30 minutes for meals.

## 🐾 Blood Sugars

It may be necessary to check the blood sugar (Chapter 7) or ketones (Chapter 5).

The test supplies we use are: _____

The supplies are kept: _____

*Please record the results of any blood or urine tests in the log book.*

Time:_____Result:_____

## 🐾 Side Trips

Please be sure that if the child is away from home, with you or with friends, extra snacks and a source of sugar are taken along.

## 🐾 Other Concerns: *Concerns that we have are:*

_____

_____

_____

_____

_____

_____

If there are any questions or if our child does not feel good or vomits, please call us or the other people listed above.  Thank you.

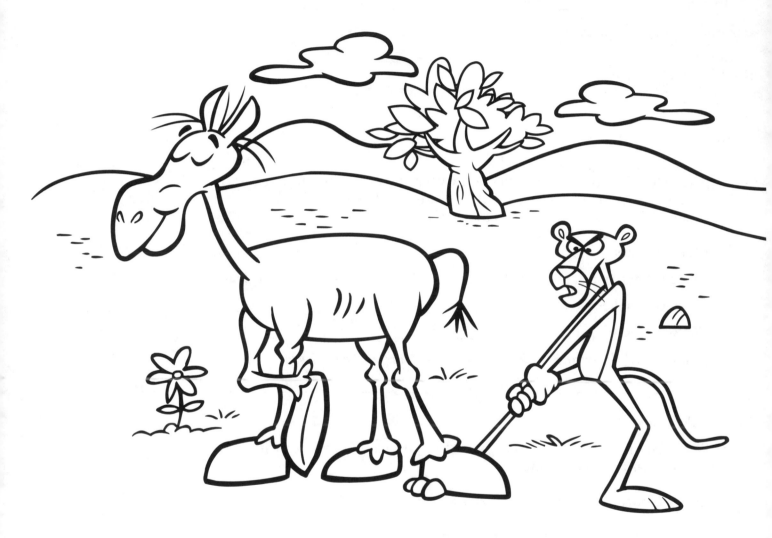

Be prepared for anything when
you're planning to camp or vacation.
Special planning is important for vacations.

# Chapter 25
# Vacations and Camp

## WHEN TRAVELING WHAT SHOULD PLANNING INCLUDE?

🐾 Insulin, blood sugar test strips, and glucagon must be kept in a plastic bag in a cooler if traveling by car. All three will spoil if they get above 90° F (3.2° C) or if they freeze.

🐾 If the meter has been in a cold place, it should be brought to room temperature before doing a blood sugar test.

🐾 Car travel may result in higher blood sugars due to less activity. Extra insulin is sometimes given.

🐾 Remember to take supplies for measuring ketones.

🐾 Insulin should be carried on airplanes and not packed in "checked-in" luggage.

🐾 Since 9/11/01, it is important with airplane travel to have a vial of insulin with the pre-printed pharmacy label on the outside of the box. The glucagon should also be left in its original container. At times of high security, it may need to be packed in a suitcase.

There have been no problems with taking insulin, insulin pumps or other diabetes supplies through x-ray security. A letter from the diabetes doctor may also be required (including his/her phone number).

🐾 Extras of everything should be carried by a second person on the plane when possible, or in a second suitcase, in case one carry-on or suitcase is lost.

🐾 Extra snacks (sugar [dextrose] tablets, granola bars, etc.) should be carried in case food is late or not available.

🐾 Time changes within the U.S. are usually not a problem, but they must be considered if going overseas (call your doctor or nurse). For insulin pumps, the time in the pump is just reset.

🐾 If activity is to be increased (playing at the beach, fishing, hiking, going to an amusement park, etc.), the insulin dose should be decreased.

# CAMP

🐾 Diabetes camp is often the first chance for a child and parents to show they can survive without each other. Most camps have doctors and nurses present so that the children are safe. Getting to know other children with diabetes who are of a similar age can be very helpful. Most of all, camp should be fun!

🐾 If going to a non-diabetes camp (or school camp/outdoor lab):

- It is essential the camp nurse and cabin counselor know about diabetes (low blood sugars and what to do, high blood sugars and what to do, illness and what to do, etc.).

- Insulin changes for camp will need to be made by the child's diabetes doctor or nurse.

- All diabetes supplies will need to be provided by the family.

- Phone numbers need to be provided to report blood sugars and receive insulin dose changes and for any emergency.

Swimming is fun . . .

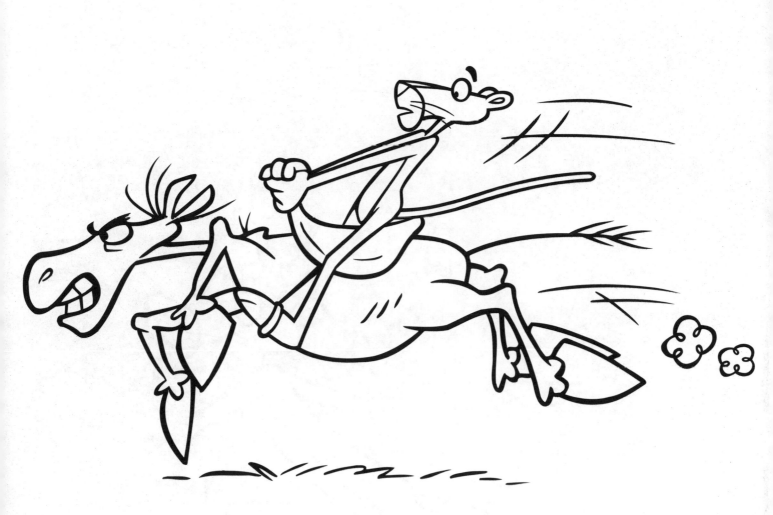

...and so is riding a horse.

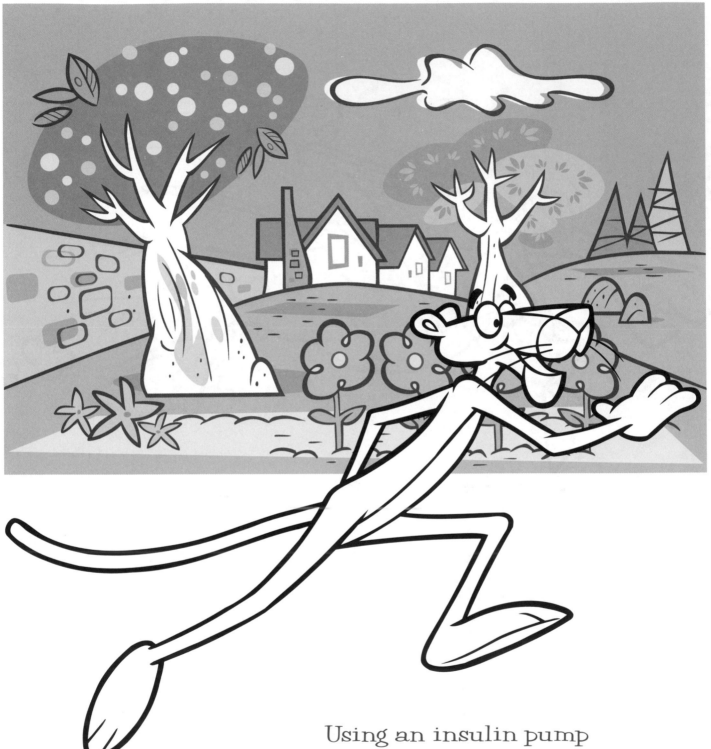

Using an insulin pump
sometimes increases one's energy.

# Chapter 26

# Use of Insulin Pumps in Diabetes Management

## THE PUMP

An insulin pump is a microcomputer (the size of a pager) that constantly provides insulin. It is important to realize that the current insulin pumps do not vary the insulin dose administered based on the blood sugar level. *Only rapid-acting insulin is used in pumps.* Pumps have become more popular in recent years. Advantages and disadvantages of pumps are discussed in Chapter 26 in the larger book, <u>Understanding Diabetes</u>. In addition, a new book <u>Understanding Insulin Pumps and Continuous Glucose Monitors</u>, is now available (see "Ordering Materials" in the back of this book).

## HOW IS INSULIN GIVEN BY THE PUMP?

🐾 The **basal** dose delivers a preset amount of insulin each hour.

🐾 A **bolus** dose is entered/given by the person wearing the pump (or by an adult) each time food is eaten or if a high blood sugar is found.

## WHAT IS INVOLVED WHEN STARTING ON A PUMP?

• The pump is more work than shots, not less. The first week (and for some, the first month) is the most difficult.

• At least four blood sugar tests must be done each day.

• Carbohydrate counting (see Chapter 12) and correction factors (Chapter 21) are usually used to determine bolus doses.

• Bolus dosages for food are best taken prior to the meal (and often 10-15 minutes before eating).

• When young children are treated with a pump, the parents are generally responsible for counting carbohydrates and giving the bolus insulin doses.

- The "smart pumps" have insulin-to-carbohydrate (I/C) ratios and correction factors programmed into them per the physician and family. Then when a blood sugar and/or grams of carbohydrate to be eaten are entered, the pump suggests an appropriate insulin dose. This dose can be given as suggested or it can be changed.

- Basal and bolus insulin doses are individualized for each person. The physician usually suggests initial basal rates.

- Close contact with the health care providers is essential.

- Our experience shows that children do well if they and their parents are both highly motivated.

- *The person with diabetes must be ready for the pump.* It must not be just the parents!

## THREE MAIN PROBLEMS SEEN WITH INSULIN "PUMPERS":

 forgetting to give bolus doses

 getting lazy and not doing at least four blood sugar tests per day

the cannula (tube) coming out from under the skin, causing blood sugars (± ketones) to rapidly rise (remember: only rapid-acting insulin is used in a pump)

When a family is ready to consider use of an insulin pump, Chapter 26 in the larger book should be read. They should then discuss the possibility with their diabetes care providers.

The person
with diabetes must
want to use the pump
(NOT just the parents).

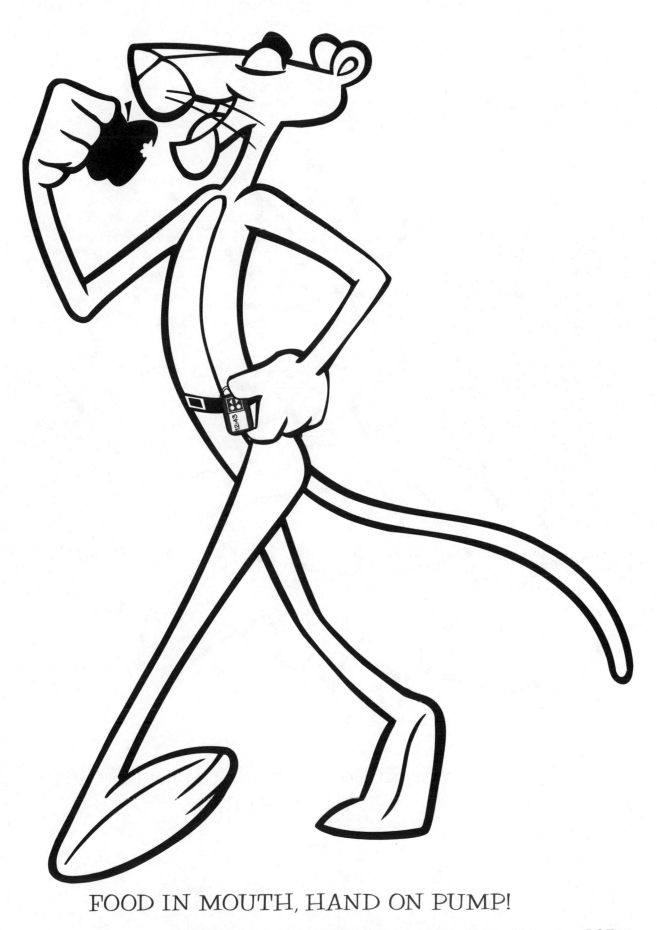

FOOD IN MOUTH, HAND ON PUMP!

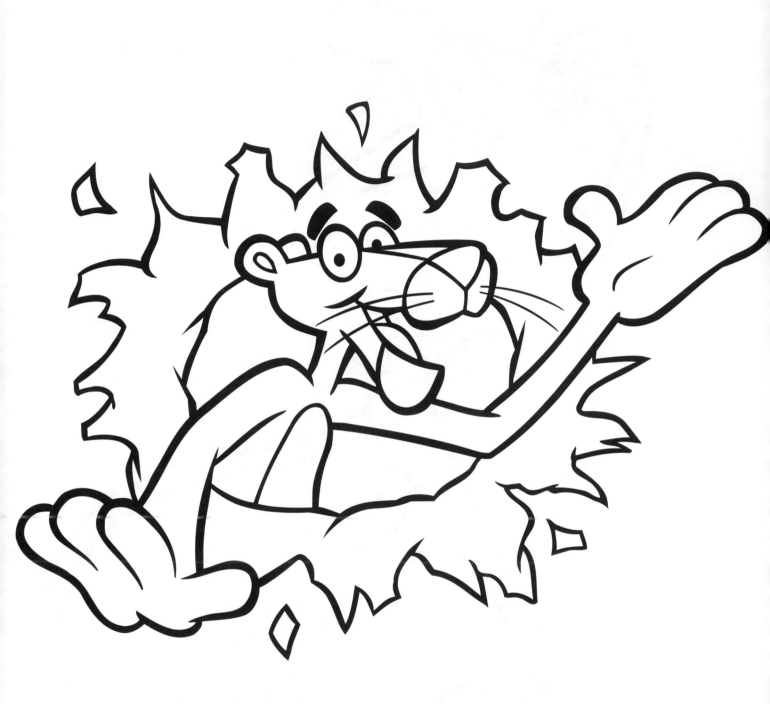

Good sugar control prior to pregnancy
is essential!

# Chapter 27
# Pregnancy and Diabetes

Pregnancy is possible for women with diabetes who do not have severe problems with complications.

## WHAT IS IMPORTANT WHEN THINKING ABOUT GETTING PREGNANT?

🐾 Pregnancy should be <u>planned</u>.

🐾 The best blood sugar control possible should be achieved before and during pregnancy. The HbA$_{1c}$ should be below 6.5%.

🐾 The risk of a miscarriage as well as birth defects in the baby are less if blood sugars are normal or near normal when the pregnancy begins.

🐾 Folic acid should be taken for three months before the pregnancy to also help prevent birth defects.

## HOW CAN THE BEST BLOOD SUGAR CONTROL BE DONE?

🐾 Intensive insulin therapy is usual during pregnancy. This includes:

- an insulin pump or frequent insulin shots

- frequent blood sugar checks (eight to ten a day)

- paying close attention to nutrition

- frequent contact with the health care team

🐾 The target values for blood sugars are lower than usual and are given in the table in Chapter 27 of <u>*Understanding Diabetes*</u>.

🐾 Clinic visits are also more often: usually every two to four weeks.

# WHAT ABOUT COMPLICATIONS AND PREGNANCY?

- Kidney damage is not a problem during pregnancy unless already present before the pregnancy. Medicines used to prevent kidney damage called "ACE-inhibitors" should not be taken during pregnancy. This medicine could cause birth defects in the baby.

- The eyes should be checked more often during pregnancy (at least every three months). If moderate damage is already present, this may get worse during pregnancy.

- Gestational diabetes is diabetes that develops as a result of the stress of the pregnancy. Regular exercise and diet are important.

  - After diagnosis, the care is like the care of a person who had diabetes prior to pregnancy.

  - Gestational diabetes usually goes away after pregnancy. There is an increased risk of developing type 2 diabetes later in life.

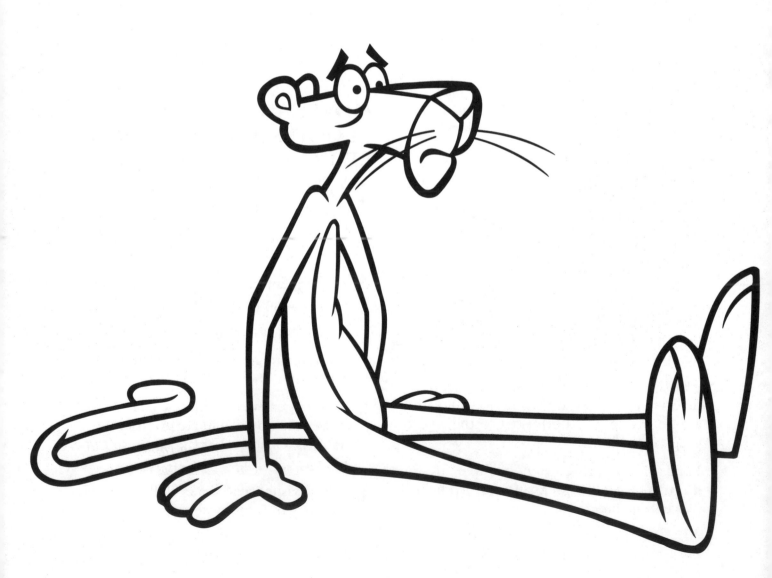

# Chapter 28
# Research and Type 1 Diabetes

This area is always changing.

## THE FIVE SUBJECTS PEOPLE ASK MOST ABOUT ARE:

**1  A cure:**

Pancreas or islet transplantation is already possible.  The problem is that the strong medicines necessary to prevent rejection can be more harmful than having diabetes.  Many new medicines are being tried, but it is still early.  Fortunately, advances are being made in the intensive management of diabetes, providing this as an alternative to surgical transplantation and a life of immunosuppression.

**2  Continuous Glucose Monitor (CGM) devices:**

Three CGM devices that will likely change diabetes management are:  the Navigator® system from Abbott Diabetes Care, the Guardian® (Paradigm®) Real Time (RT) system from Medtronic MiniMed and the DexCom™ STS™.  All have a small sensor with a "needle" worn under the skin that transmits subcutaneous glucose levels every one to five minutes (by radio telemetry) to a receiver or insulin pump.  However, none of them at this time controls insulin output by an insulin pump.  All have alarms for low and high glucose readings.  It is likely these CGM devices will bring about the "third era" of diabetes management:

I)       Urine sugar testing

II)      Blood sugar testing

III)     CGM (the "third era")

A new book, _Understanding Insulin Pumps and Continuous Glucose Monitors_ is now available (see "Ordering Materials" in the back of this book).

**Prevention of type 1 diabetes (see www.diabetestrialnet.org):**

- Several trials are currently under way.

- In the U.S., people can call 1-800-425-8361 to find out where to go for a free TrialNet antibody screening. This area is moving very rapidly.

- Three biochemical islet cell antibodies (Chapter 3) are being used to determine if the autoimmune process has begun.

- Prevention trials are now focused on:

  ~ preventing the autoimmune process from starting

  ~ reversing the antibodies

  ~ stopping further damage after diabetes has been diagnosed

- It is likely that prevention will come before a safe cure.

**Prevention of type 2 diabetes:**

- This has already been shown to be possible.

- It involves eating less, exercising more, and losing weight.

- It is discussed in Chapter 4 of "Understanding Diabetes."

**Prevention of complications:**

- Diabetes complications of the eye and kidney are decreasing through attention being paid to the following:

  ~ better sugar control

  ~ blood pressure control

  ~ not smoking

  ~ yearly eye exams and urine microalbumin tests - essential after three years of diabetes in people age 12 years or older (see Chapter 22). Families may need to help remind their diabetes care provider to make sure these tests are done.

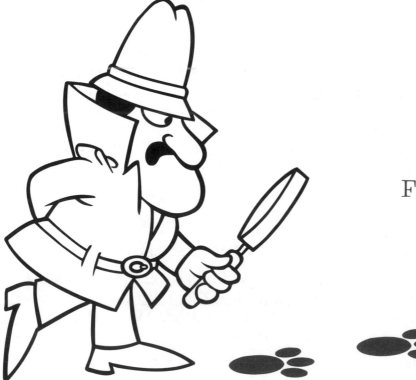

Finding the cure

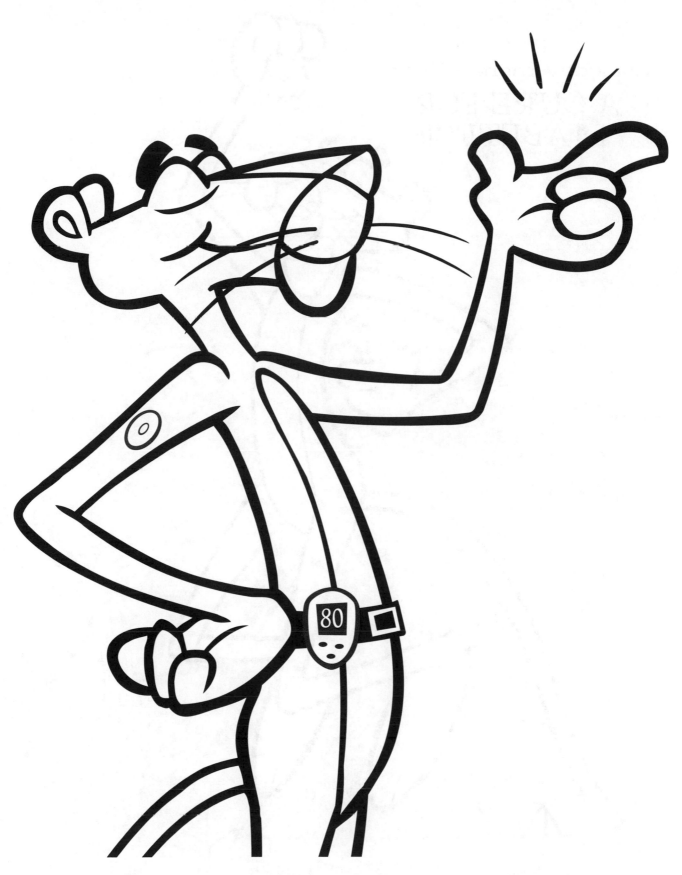

Continuous Glucose Monitoring is here!

Someday there will be

# A CURE FOR DIABETES!

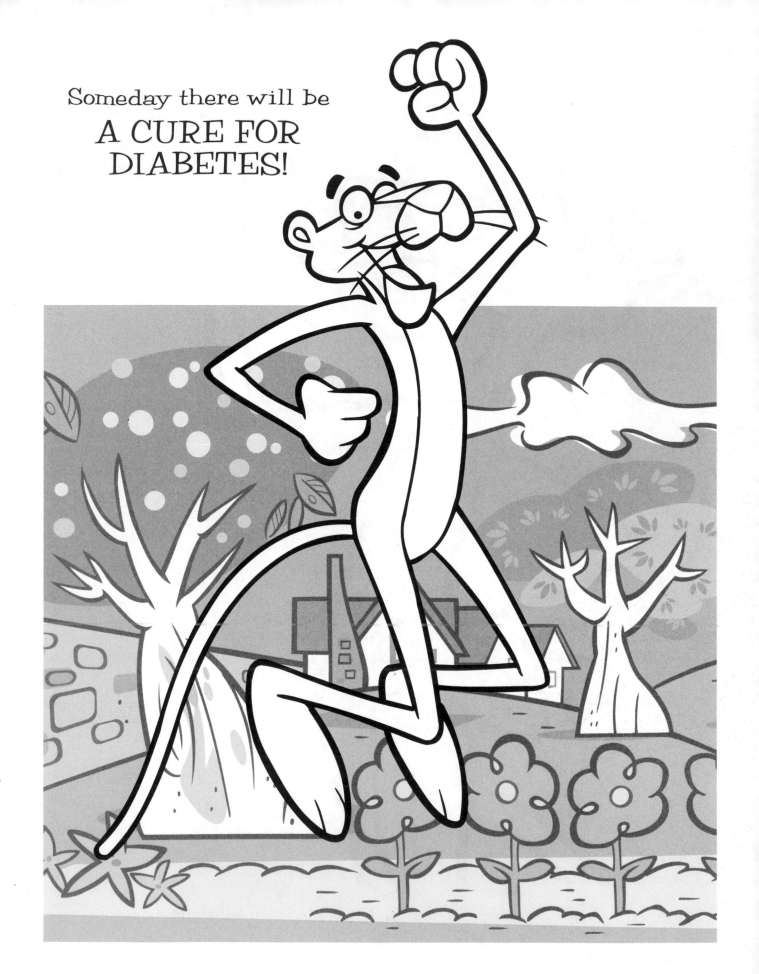

H. PETER CHASE, MD is the past Executive and Clinical Director of the Barbara Davis Center for Childhood Diabetes in Denver, CO.  In addition, he is a Professor of Pediatrics at the University of Colorado Health Sciences Center in Aurora, CO.

Dr. Chase received his education at the University of Wisconsin in Madison, WI.  He completed his internship and residency at the University of Utah and Stanford University.  A fellowship in Endocrinology and metabolism (Stanford and the University of Colorado) was followed by research at the National Institute of Health.  He has since been a faculty member of the University of Colorado.  He has been a principal investigator in the multi-center NIH – funded studies of Diabetes Research in Children Network (DIRECNET) and the Type 1 Diabetes/TrialNet prevention studies.  He currently has two research grants from the Juvenile Diabetes Research Foundation (JDRF).

Dr. Chase has received many honors, including the Outstanding Physician Clinician in Diabetes award from the American Diabetes Association, a Lifetime Achievement Award from JDRF and the Ross Award for Outstanding Research in Pediatrics.  He has authored over 250 research papers and 50 textbook chapters.  In addition to this synopsis <u>A First Book for Understanding Diabetes</u>, the larger 11th Edition of <u>Understanding Diabetes</u> follows the same outline of chapters.

Financial Disclosures:  Dr Chase has no current financial disclosures.

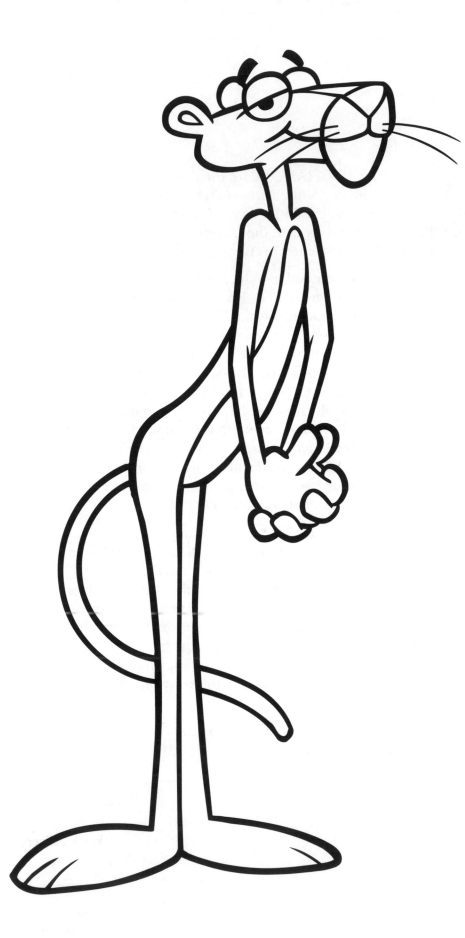

# ORDERING MATERIALS

**Additional copies** of *A First Book for Understanding Diabetes*
as well as other diabetes informational material may be ordered by using this form,
by calling the Children's Diabetes Foundation at 303-863-1200 or 800-695-2873, by e-mailing
cdfcares@childrensdiabetesfdn.org, or by visiting our website at
**ChildrensDiabetesFoundation.org**

## Children's Diabetes Foundation
### 777 Grant Street • Suite 302 • Denver, CO 80203

Name_____

Address_____

City, State, ZIP_____

Phone_____Email_____

| Quantity | Item | Price | Total |
|---|---|---|---|
| | *A First Book for Understanding Diabetes* Presents the essentials from *Understanding Diabetes* in synopsis-fashion. | $10.00 | |
| | *Un Primer Libro Para Entender La Diabetes* Spanish version of *A First Book for Understanding Diabetes* | $10.00 | |
| | *Understanding Diabetes* – The Pink Panther Book 11th Edition | $25.00 | |
| | *Understanding Insulin Pumps and Continuous Glucose Monitors* First Edition | $15.00 | |
| | **VIDEO: Managing Diabetic Hypoglycemia** Offers people with diabetes of all ages and backgrounds practical suggestions for how they can manage and prevent low blood sugar during a busy, productive day. | $20.00 | |
| | | TOTAL | |

☐ Please include me on the Children's Diabetes Foundation mailing list.

☐ Check enclosed payable to: CDF at Denver

☐ VISA ☐ MasterCard ☐ Discover ☐ AmEx

Card # _____ Exp. Date _____

Signature _____

All orders must be paid in full before delivery.
Books are mailed USPS or Ground UPS. Allow one to three weeks for delivery.

Canadian and Foreign Purchasers:
Please include sufficient funds to equal U.S. currency exchange rates.

For quantity order pricing and additional information call 303-863-1200 or 800-695-2873
or visit our website at: www.ChildrensDiabetesFoundation.org

# WEBSITES

Barbara Davis Center for Childhood Diabetes
University of Colorado Denver
Mail Stop A140
P.O. Box 6511
Aurora, CO 80045
303-724-2323 · Fax 303-724-6779
www.BarbaraDavisCenter.org

Children's Diabetes Foundation at Denver, Colorado
www.ChildrensDiabetesFoundation.org

Children With Diabetes
www.ChildrenwithDiabetes.com

Juvenile Diabetes Research Foundation
www.jdrf.org

American Diabetes Association
www.diabetes.org